The *In Practice* Handbooks

Equine
Practice 2

Edited by E. Boden
Executive Editor, *In Practice*

Baillière Tindall

LONDON   PHILADELPHIA   TORONTO   SYDNEY   TOKYO

Baillière Tindall   24–28 Oval Road
W. B. Saunders   London NW1 7DX

The Curtis Center
Independence Square West
Philadelphia, PA 19106-3399, USA

55 Horner Avenue
Toronto, Ontario, M8Z 4X6, Canada

Harcourt Brace Jovanovich Group
(Australia) Pty Ltd
30–52 Smidmore Street
Marrickville
NSW 2204, Australia

Harcourt Brace Jovanovich Japan Inc
Ichibancho Central Building
22-1 Ichibancho
Chiyoda-ku, Tokyo 102, Japan

Typeset by Photo·graphics, Honiton, Devon
Printed and bound in Hong Kong by Dah Hua Printing Press Co., Ltd.

A catalogue record for this book is available from
the British Library

ISBN 0-7020-1686-1

Equine Practice 2

Withdrawn

The *In Practice* Handbooks Series

Series Editor: Edward Boden

Past and present members of *In Practice* Editorial Board

Titles in print:
Feline Practice
Canine Practice
Equine Practice
Bovine Practice
Sheep and Goat Practice
Swine Practice
Small Animal Practice
Poultry Practice
Equine Practice 2

Contents

Contributors

A. Barr, University of Bristol, School of Veterinary Science, Langford House, Langford, Bristol, UK

C. Brown, Large Animal Clinical Sciences, Michigan State University, East Lansing, Michigan 48864, USA

D. Cuddeford, Royal (Dick) School of Veterinary Studies, Veterinary Field Station, Easter Bush, Nr Roslin, Midlothian, UK

D. R. Ellis, Reynolds House, 166 High Street, Newmarket, Suffolk, UK

R. Ellis, Veterinary Surgery, Beulah, Llanwrtyd Wells, Powys, UK

R. Eustace, The Laminitis Clinic, University of Bristol, Veterinary Field Station, Langford House, Langford, Bristol, UK

C. Gibbs, University of Bristol, School of Veterinary Science, Langford House, Langford, Bristol, UK

T. Greet, Rossdale & Partners, Beaufort Cottage Stables & Laboratories, High Street, Newmarket, Suffolk, UK

G. Lane, Senior Lecturer in Surgery, University of Bristol, School of Veterinary Science, Langford House, Langford, Bristol, UK

T. Mair, John McCaig & Eryl V Davies, Veterinary Practitioners, 123 Commercial Road, Paddock Wood, Kent, UK

E. Milne, Royal (Dick) School of Veterinary Studies, Department of Veterinary Medicine, Veterinary Field Station, Easter Bush, Nr Roslin, Midlothian, UK

T. Mullaney, Animal Health Diagnostic Laboratory, PO Box 30076, Lansing, Michigan 48909, USA

G. A. Munroe, University of Glasgow, Veterinary School, Bearsden Road, Bearsden, Glasgow, UK

S. W. Ricketts, Rossdale & Partners, Beaufort Cottage Stables & Laboratories, High Street, Newmarket, Suffolk UK

S. Robertson, Department of Small Animal Clinical Science, Michigan State University, East Lansing, Michigan 48864, USA

L. Young, Department of Veterinary Anaesthesia, Faculty of Veterinary Science, University of Liverpool, Liverpool, UK

Foreword

In Practice was started in 1979 as a clinical supplement to *The Veterinary Record*. Its carefully chosen, highly illustrated articles specially commissioned from leaders in their field were aimed specifically at the practitioner. In the form of "opinionated reviews", they have proved extremely popular with experienced veterinarians and students alike. The editorial board, chaired for the first 10 years by Professor James Armour, was particularly concerned to emphasize differential diagnosis.

In response to consistent demand, articles from *In Practice*, updated and revised by the authors, are now published in convenient handbook form. Each book deals with a particular species or group of related animals.

E. Boden

CHAPTER 1

Standing Chemical Restraint in the Horse

GRAHAM MUNROE AND LESLEY YOUNG

INTRODUCTION

Chemical restraint is an invaluable technique in equine clinical practice. The introduction of safer, effective and more reliable drugs has allowed procedures that previously could only be undertaken under general anaesthesia, to be safely completed in the standing horse. Thus, the disadvantages associated with general anaesthesia and prolonged recumbency in this species can often all be avoided. Standing chemical restraint is of particular benefit in radiography, biopsy collection, endoscopy and minor surgical techniques.

The amount of chemical restraint required will vary depending on the individual horse, the environment and the procedure to be undertaken. In addition, the depth of sedation/analgesia will vary enormously according to the drugs or combinations being used. Local anaesthesia is a powerful adjunct to all forms of chemical restraint, whether regional, infiltrative or epidural techniques are employed.

In all cases, it is preferable that the horse is kept in quiet surroundings before drug administration and while sedation is allowed to develop. The injection of the agents must take place quickly and efficiently. For most drugs the intravenous route is the most rapidly effective and reliable. After intravenous administration sedation can take in excess of five minutes to develop fully and, if intravenous acepromazine is used alone, a further 20 minutes is required. Generally, at least 25 minutes will be required for peak sedation to develop after intramuscular administration of most drugs.

Before any central nervous system depressant drug is given to a horse or pony, the patient should be carefully examined for any pre-existing conditions that may be exacerbated by the use of the drug, or that may potentiate the agent's side effects. The results of this evaluation must be married with the clinician's knowledge of the available sedative/tranquillizers such that the upshot of the process is the "right drug for the right job".

TRANQUILLIZERS

PHENOTHIAZINES

Tranquillizers for use in equine practice are now almost exclusively restricted to the phenothiazine group, specifically acepromazine maleate (Table 1.1). Classically, the phenothiazines are said to produce a state of stoical indifference to the surroundings in a wide variety of species. This type of effect is often sufficient to calm a nervous animal for minimally invasive procedures such as clipping or loading. Unfortunately, while a proportion of horses will be profoundly sedated by a given dose of acepromazine, other individuals will be seemingly unaffected or very easily aroused.

Acepromazine is a potent alpha-adrenergic blocker, causing dose-dependent vasodilation and hypotension. Thus conditions in which there may be any suspicion of cardiovascular compromise or hypovolaemia represent absolute contraindications to its use.

All phenothiazines, but specifically acepromazine, have also been associated with priapism (persistent penile erection, not associated with sexual stimulation) and paraphimosis (protrusion of the flaccid penis through the preputial orifice) (Fig. 1.1). Although early support and medical management can be effective, in some instances prolonged exposure of the penis and subsequent severe trauma and damage have

Table 1.1 Sedatives/tranquillizers used for standing restraint.

Drug	Manufacturer	Cost*(£)
Acepromazine maleate		
ACP injection, 10 mg/ml	C-Vet	
20 ml vial (POM)		
0.05–0.10 mg/kg im (slow iv)	Bk Vet Products	<1
ACP tablets, 10 mg and 25 mg	C-Vet	
1000 (POM)		<1
10–20 tablets		
Xylazine		
Rompun Dry Substance 5 × 500 mg +	Bayer	
Solvent (POM)		
0.8–1.0 mg/kg iv		11–20
2.4–3.0 mg/kg im		31–40
Anased 100 mg/ml 10 ml vial (POM)	BK Vet Products	
0.5–1.1 mg/kg iv		1–10
2.2 mg/kg im		21–30
Detomidine hydrochloride		
Domosedan 10 mg/ml	Norden	
5 ml and 20 ml vials (POM)	Laboratories	
10–20 µg/kg iv/im		1–10
Romifidine		
Sedivet 10mg/ml	Boehringer	1–10
20 ml vials (POM)	Ingelheim	
50–100 µg/kg im/iv		

*Cost refers to lowest dose rate for a 500 kg horse using the cheapest purchasable quantity (January 1992 prices)
iv intravenously
im intramuscularly

necessitated penile amputation and even euthanasia; in most reported cases acepromazine maleate was used in conjunction with etorphine in the neuroleptic mixture Large Animal Immobilon (C-Vet). In some, however, phenothiazines were used alone, usually by the intravenous route. Thus, it is recommended that these drugs are not used in breeding stallions.

Acepromazine may be administered by the intramuscular or the intravenous route. It is doubtful whether, when used alone, the intravenous route offers any significant advantage over intramuscular administration, because sedation is slow

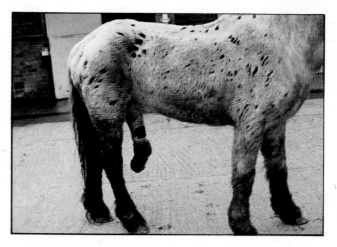

Fig. 1.1
Swollen, paralysed
penis showing severe
secondary trauma in
a horse given
acepromazine.

to develop in both cases. In contrast to most other agents the
drug is also available in tablet form.

BENZODIAZEPINES

The use of benzodiazepines, which are known to have
anxiolytic, anamnestic and tranquillizing properties in
humans, has been described in the adult horse. The results,
however, can be unpredictable and unmanageable ataxia
frequently results from profound somatic muscle relaxation.
This has tended to restrict their use in adult horses to adjuncts
in anaesthetic induction techniques. However, the remarkable
cardiovascular and respiratory stability of both diazepam and
midazolam has made these very useful drugs in both neonatal
and critically ill foals, where ataxia and recumbency are easily
managed.

SEDATIVE HYPNOTICS (Table 1.1)

ALPHA-ADRENORECEPTOR AGONISTS

The recent advances in alpha-adrenoreceptor pharmacology
have produced three drugs, xylazine, detomidine and romifidine, that have revolutionized standing chemical restraint in

the horse (Fig. 1.2). The drugs produce generalized central nervous system depression accompanied by muscle relaxation and some analgesia. The drugs also produce complex cardio-vascular effects, bradydysrythmias being frequently observed. Generally, these potentially deleterious effects are well toler-ated in normal animals. However, care should be taken in older or debilitated animals because the effects may be profound. Other side effects include localized muscle tremors, patchy or widespread sweating and increased frequency of urination.

It must be emphasized that, despite the appearance of profound sedation, many horses are capable of violent avoidance behaviour when a painful stimulus is applied, and maintain the ability to deliver a well aimed kick. Thus when contemplating painful manipulations, caution should always be displayed and the drugs should be used in conjunction with local anaesthetic techniques and, or, combined with an opiate (see later).

CHLORAL HYDRATE

The popularity of chloral hydrate as an intravenously adminis-tered sedative/hypnotic in horses has declined enormously as more convenient and reliable drugs have become available. Rarely, however, it may still be used by the oral route

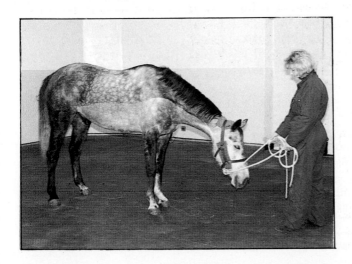

Fig. 1.2
Adult horse sedated
with a 10 μg/kg dose
of detomidine.

to facilitate the handling of a particularly unruly horse. Unfortunately when dissolved in water the drug has an unpleasant taste and it may take up to 24 hours before the horse will drink the solution. It has been suggested that the drug may be more palatable when mixed with a small meal.

OPIOIDS/NARCOTIC ANALGESICS (Table 1.2)

The opioids/narcotic analgesics interact with specific opioid receptors within the central nervous system. Their clinical effects are diverse and include analgesia, sedation, euphoria, disorientation and dysphoria. In addition, other body systems can also be affected, including control of gut motility and depression of respiration.

In general, the horse tends to exhibit the excitatory effects more readily than most other species, particularly when the more potent opiates are used in healthy, pain-free subjects. Although the tendency for excitement is much reduced when the drugs are used in horses already in pain, it is recommended that analgesic doses of the potent opiates (morphine, metha-

Table 1.2 Analgesics used for standing restraint.

Drug	Manufacturer	Cost*(£)
Pethidine hydrochloride Pethidine, 50 ml bottle (POM) Schedule 2 50 mg/ml 2–5 mg/kg im	Arnolds Veterinary Products	1–10
Butorphanol tartrate Torbugesic injection, 10 and 50 ml bottle (POM) 10 mg/ml 0.1 mg/kg iv	C-Vet	1–10
Morphine sulphate BP Morphine injection, 2 ml vials POM Schedule 2, 30 mg/ml 0.1 mg/kg im	Evans	1–10
Methadone sulphate BP Physeptone 30 mg POM Schedule 2, 10 mg/ml 0.05 mg/kg im	Wellcome	

*See Table 1.1. iv intravenously
im intramuscularly

done, pethidine) be administered by the intramuscular route. This does not apply to butorphanol which can be given in full doses intravenously without causing excitement.

Respiratory depression is also a known side effect of opiate administration. However, when the drugs are used in conscious horses, including when combined with a sedative/tranquillizer, the respiratory depression produced is usually well tolerated since the animal remains standing.

CONTROLLED DRUG REGULATIONS

The possibility of opioid dependence in humans has led to most of the commonly used opiates (including morphine, pethidine, methadone and papaveretum) being classified as Schedule 2 drugs under The Misuse of Drugs Act (1983). In practice, if these drugs are to be used, an up to date, comprehensive record of their supply and each individual dispatch must be kept available for examination for two full years after the final entry is made. Additionally, the drugs must be carried within a locked box (NB: for the purpose of the Act, merely carrying the drugs loose in a locked car is not considered to be acceptable). Failure to adhere to the provisions of the Act render the veterinary surgeon liable to prosecution. As yet the synthetic opiod, butorphanol, is not subject to control, which may certainly account for some of its popularity.

DRUG COMBINATIONS

When opioids are administered alone to healthy, pain-free subjects they do not cause sedation *per se* and may even cause stimulation. However, when they are used in combination with the aforementioned sedatives/tranquillizers, marked synergy occurs between the two groups of drugs. This results in greatly increased sedation and marked analgesia for more painful manipulations. The addition of a tranquillizer or a sedative will often ameliorate the excitatory effects of the opioid. Because only small doses of individual drugs are employed, recovery times are not significantly altered; neither are the combinations associated with an increased degree of cardiovascular depression.

A plethora of sedative/tranquillizer/narcotic combinations have been used successfully for standing sedation in the horse. A selection of the more popular combinations are included in Table 1.3. Use of the alpha-2 agonist, detomidine, with the synthetic opioid, butorphanol is very popular, providing profound sedation, adequate for most procedures. The ataxia produced by this combination can be inconvenient, particularly if the manipulation is to be performed on the limbs. Early work with the newly developed alpha-2 adrenergic agonist, romifidine, suggests that the ataxia produced is less pronounced when romifidine replaces detomidine in this combination.

Table 1.3 Intravenous sedative combinations in the horse.

Combinations	Dose rate	Comments
Xylazine	0.5 mg/kg	Rapid onset
Butorphanol	0.025 mg/kg	Dependable
		Deep standing sedation
		Some ataxia
Detomidine	10 µg/kg	As above
Butorphanol	0.025 mg/kg	
Romifidine	50 µg/kg	As above but less ataxia
Butorphanol	0.025 mg/kg	
Xylazine	0.4 mg/kg	Good standing sedation with little ataxia
Acepromazine	0.05 mg/kg	No somatic analgesia
Xylazine	0.2 mg/kg	As above
Acepromazine	0.05 mg/kg	Plus somatic analgesia
Pethidine	0.4 mg/kg	Equivalent to xylazine/detomidine + butorphanol
Acepromazine	0.05 mg/kg	Short duration
Methadone	0.1 mg/kg	Moderate sedation/analgesia
Xylazine	0.5 mg/kg	As above
Methadone	0.1 mg/kg	

NB: Only pethidine and butorphanol are licensed for use in the horse. Unpublished research suggests that the drugs can be administered simultaneously and mixed. All drugs should be administered by slow intravenous injection.

SPECIAL SITUATIONS

PREGNANCY

The use of sedative/tranquillizers in pregnant mares is often a cause for concern. Very few of these drugs have been tested in mares for teratogenic or abortigenic effects and data from other species cannot always be applied. Particular times for concern are the periods of organogenesis (first two months) and the latter stages of pregnancy.

As a result of interaction with uterine alpha-2 receptors, xylazine has been shown to stimulate uterine contraction in the bovine, and may cause abortion in the third trimester of pregnancy. Detomidine, which also acts via alpha-2 receptors could have similar effects. Consequently, xylazine and detomidine have both been contraindicated in the latter stages of pregnancy. However, recent work using detomidine through-out all stages of gestation, although based on small numbers of mares, did suggest that repeated administrations of the drug did not have specific adverse effects on the pregnancy or the fetus. This would support clinical experiences of using the drug in pregnant mares.

Acepromazine has no specific contraindications and although like most sedative drugs it will readily cross the placenta, it has minimal cardiovascular and central nervous system depressive effects on the fetus. The opioids also cross the placenta and in view of their ability to depress respiration in the fetus, they should be used with great caution around the time of parturition. Specific opiate antagonists, such as naloxone, will be useful if a foal is delivered and transplacental opiate-induced respiratory depression is suspected.

Clinicians should evaluate the possible benefits and dangers of using all these drugs in pregnant mares on an individual basis and inform owners as to the possible consequences.

FOALS

Healthy neonatal foals lack disciplinary training and are often more active than adults. Thus, a procedure which is relatively simple in the adult may require sedation or even general anaesthesia in the foal. Physical restraint, especially by experienced stud personnel, can be useful but the use of vigorous manual restraint for prolonged periods is contraindicated. Besides the compromise to the proposed technique there are very real problems of injury and stress to the foal.

Unfortunately there is relatively little published information on sedation and anaesthesia in the foal. In addition, the pharmacokinetics of most drugs in the neonate differ significantly from those in the adult. However, with caution, most agents used in adults can be used in older foals and in healthy neonates. Acepromazine is perhaps the least useful because its duration tends to be prolonged, promoting hypothermia and hypotension, while generally the sedation produced by moderate doses of this drug are insufficient for restraint. Xylazine is commonly used and has several advantages over the phenothiazine derivatives. It causes profound sedation, has a rapid onset and dose-dependent duration of action. It is best given intravenously at a dose rate of 0.3 to 1.0 mg/kg and provides 15 to 40 minutes of sedation. This can be deepened easily to the stage of recumbency, if required, by the use of intravenous morphine (0.3 to 0.6 mg/kg) or butorphanol (20 to 40 µg/kg). These combinations will provide restraint adequate for radiography, cast application, endoscopy and in conjunction with local anaesthesia for minor surgery.

The effects of detomidine have recently been studied in the foal and it has been shown to provide similar, reliable sedation with a dose-dependent duration of action (10 to 40 µg/kg). Although the drug appears to be well tolerated in the normal foal, in view of the drug's high potency and commercial formulation (10 mg/ml) the risk of involuntary overdose to neonates is much higher and great caution is advised.

TRANSPORTING INJURED EQUINES

Sedatives, particularly those with strong analgesic effects, can be useful in the transportation of animals with fractures or severe soft tissue injuries. Of equal importance is stabilization and support of the fracture or injury by application of a cast, splint or bandage-splint combination. If movement of the injury is prevented by splinting, much of the associated pain and distress will be ameliorated and further deterioration of the orthopaedic condition will be prevented. Parenterally administered analgesia will never substitute for good first aid. The use of analgesics without sedative effects is desirable because any ataxia may further damage the injury, particularly when travelling. The opiates, such as pethidine, methadone or morphine, can be useful and they can be supplemented or replaced by the non-steroidal anti-inflammatory drugs, e.g. phenylbutazone. Acepromazine should be avoided in animals after acute trauma in view of its tendency to produce hypotension in the face of possible haemorrhage.

COLIC

Examination of an animal suffering severe abdominal pain represents a major challenge. A detailed clinical examination to evaluate both the cardiovascular and gastrointestinal tract of the horse is crucial. A rectal examination is mandatory and in many cases the animal must be restrained for the passage of a nasogastric tube. If the animal is violent and facilities for restraint are not available, chemical means may be employed to aid examinations and minimize danger to personnel. Xylazine is undoubtedly the drug of choice in this situation, the intravenous route being preferred. Frequently, 0.2 to 0.4 mg/kg is sufficient to allow a rectal examination. An additional 0.2 mg/kg may be administered if the initial sedation is not sufficient. At low dose rates the drug is short acting and will not mask the development of clinical signs which might indicate that surgical intervention is required.

For horses that are unresponsive to xylazine alone, the intravenous administration of 25 to 50 μg/kg of butorphanol is usually sufficient to transiently calm even the most violent case of colic. This synthetic opioid has been shown experimentally to produce visceral analgesia in the horse. Clinical experience also shows the drug to be of great benefit in the horse with colic. In addition, the spasmolytic properties of pethidine also facilitate excellent visceral analgesia. It is rapidly absorbed from intramuscular sites, thus 1 g of pethidine intramuscularly represents a very inexpensive alternative to butorphanol. As a result of its prolonged duration of action and increased potency, detomidine should be used only with great caution in this situation.

If intravenous injection is impossible, both xylazine and detomidine can be administered by the intramuscular route. Of the two drugs, detomidine is probably the most effectively absorbed from this site. It is suggested that 1.5 to two times the equivalent intravenous dose of detomidine is required for similar effects, while three times the equivalent dose of xylazine may be needed.

The alpha-adrenergic blocking effect of acepromazine maleate renders it completely unsuitable for use in cases of equine colic.

DONKEYS

Very little specific research has been carried out into drug pharmacokinetics in the donkey. Fortunately most drugs and drug combinations at standard dose rates have been used clinically with good consistent results. One occasionally reported side effect of detomidine has been an increased incidence of facial/head oedema. This is rapidly resolved by elevating the head.

ACKNOWLEDGEMENTS

The authors would like to express their thanks to Dr J. E. Cox of the Department of Equine Studies, University of Liverpool, for kindly lending the photograph depicting penile paralysis and to Mr D. Bartram for his help in reading the manuscript.

REFERENCES AND FURTHER READING

Hall, L. W. & Clarke, K. W. (1983). *Veterinary Anaesthesia*, 8th edn, p. 203. London, Baillière Tindall.

Jordan, W. J. (1986). Surgery including Restraint and General Anaesthesia. In *Professional Handbook of the Donkey* (ed E. Svendsen), p. 101. Devon, The Donkey Sanctuary.

Klein, L. (1985). *Equine Practice* **1**, 77.

Pearson, H. & Weaver, M. Q. B. (1978). *Equine Veterinary Journal,* **10**, 85.

Code of practice for storage and dispensing of medicines by veterinary surgeons. (1991). London, British Veterinary Association.

CHAPTER 2

The Barren Mare: Diagnosis, Prognosis, Prophylaxis and Treatment for Genital Abnormality

SIDNEY RICKETTS

INTRODUCTION

To aim for maximal breeding efficiency, all barren mares should receive a thorough gynaecological examination after the end of the breeding season but before they go into winter anoestrus, e.g. in September, with the aim of:

(1) Making a diagnosis of genital abnormality, if one is present.
(2) Making a provisional breeding prognosis based on the diagnosis.
(3) Formulating and carrying out a logical treatment programme if indicated.
(4) Assessing the response to treatment after a period of rest.
(5) Making a more accurate breeding prognosis based on diagnosis and assessment of response.
(6) Repeating or substituting alternative treatment if response is unsatisfactory, until improvement occurs or retirement is recommended.

(7) Allowing an extended period of rest before the next breeding season.

Without this approach many mares enter the next breeding season with persistent genital abnormalities which require definition, treatment, reassessment and recovery, delaying mating and wasting valuable time. The necessarily shortened recovery periods are less satisfactory.

An accurate diagnosis is, as always, a pre-requisite to prognosis, treatment and successful management. This requires a detailed logical investigatory approach, using all appropriate diagnostic techniques, designed to formulate a differential diagnosis and leading if possible, to a definitive diagnosis.

DIAGNOSIS

A detailed general and gynaecological/obstetrical history should be taken from the mare owner, stud manager and, or, groom.

AGE

A barren maiden mare, in contrast to an aged multiparous mare, is unlikely to be suffering from chronic degenerative endometrial disease, but may have a fundamental genetic abnormality definable by chromosome analysis.

TYPE

A barren thoroughbred mare has probably visited a stallion annually since she was a four year old. A barren hunter may have had only the occasional visit, when management may have been less than satisfactory.

GENERAL VETERINARY HISTORY

An equine herpesvirus I or "strangles" outbreak or an injury may have reduced mating opportunities.

GYNAECOLOGICAL/OBSTETRICAL HISTORY

Veterinary gynaecological management

The mare may not have been examined and appropriate mating opportunities and, or, genital abnormalities may have been missed.

Cyclical and mating history

The mare who does not "show" well to the teaser may have missed mating opportunities. The mare who "short cycles" may have persistent acute endometritis.

Pertinent gynaecological syndromes

Historical data may explain current fertility problems and may lead to specific pathways for investigations, e.g. traumatic parturition (cervical injury), venereal disease (missed mating opportunities), repeated pregnancy failure (chronic endometrial disease) and recurrent acute endometritis (uterine immune incompetence).

PHYSICAL EXAMINATION

A general physical examination should be made for signs of conditions which may affect reproductive function/efficiency. General health and condition may be relevant. Malnutrition, emaciation/cachexia or persistent pain, e.g. lameness, can inhibit normal ovarian cyclic activity.

GYNAECOLOGICAL EXAMINATIONS

These should be made under relaxed and clean conditions, with the mare adequately restrained, ideally in stocks (Fig. 2.1). The genital organs should be examined in a logical order, i.e. from vulva to ovaries.

Vulva/perineum

Discharges

A vulval discharge may be a sign of genital or urinary abnormality (Fig. 2.2).

Perineal conformation

In thoroughbred mares and less commonly other types of mare, pneumovagina with or without faecal contamination may lead to recurrent acute endometritis (Fig. 2.3). Pneumovagina may be treated by Caslick's vulvoplasty (Fig. 2.4) or Pouret's perineal reconstruction operation (Fig. 2.5). Vulval

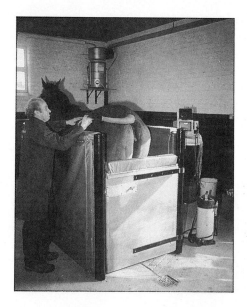

Fig. 2.1
Stocks provide adequate restraint for examination.

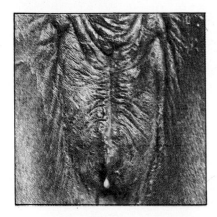

Fig. 2.2
Vulval discharge may be a sign of genital or urinary abnormality.

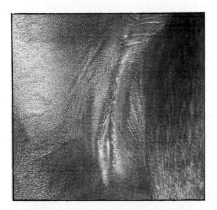

Fig. 2.3
Pneumovagina may lead to recurrent acute endometritis.

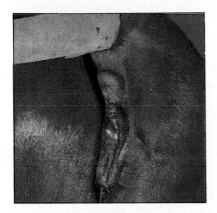

Fig. 2.4
Caslick's vulvoplasty.

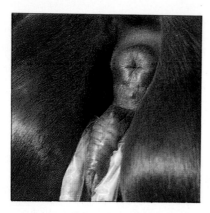

Fig. 2.5
Pouret's perineal reconstruction operation.

injury may result in incompetent lip closure, which may lead to pneumovagina, and therefore these injuries must be treated by careful surgical repair.

Clitoral and vestibular swabs

Swabs should be collected to screen for the potential disease-producing bacteria *Taylorella equigenitalis, Pseudomonas aeruginosa* and *Klebsiella pneumoniae*.

Swabs may be taken from discharges, if present, or routinely from the area of the urethral opening, in the vestibule, the clitoral fossa and the clitoral sinuses (using narrow-tipped swabs) (Fig. 2.6). Swabs should be placed immediately into Amies charcoal transport medium and transported to a

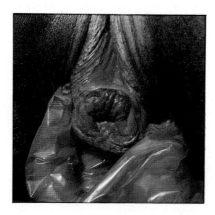

Fig. 2.6
Swabs may be taken from the area of the urethral opening, in the vestibule, the clitoral fossa and the clitoral sinuses.

laboratory experienced in performing these examinations, as soon as possible and within five days of sampling.

T. equigenitalis may be harboured in the smegma contained in the clitorial sinuses. Treatment is to remove the smegma of the fossa and sinuses with water and chlorhexidine surgical scrub, followed by packing with 2 per cent nitrofurazone ointment. Persistently intractable cases may require clitoral sinusectomy. Following these treatments, an actively growing bacterial broth made from contaminant microflora, grown in the laboratory from clitoral swabs taken from normal mares, may be applied to the clitoral area to discourage recolonization with *P. aeruginosa* or *K. pneumoniae*.

P. aeruginosa and *K. pneumoniae* may both be harboured in the clitoral fossa and, or, sinuses and sometimes the urethral opening, associated with urinary infection. Treatment is to remove all smegma with plain water and then to treat with gentamicin cream or, in the case of *P. aeruginosa*, 1 per cent aqueous silver nitrate, as a dessicant. Persistently intractable cases may require clitorectomy. Following this, an actively growing bacterial contaminant broth culture may be applied to the clitoral area to encourage early recolonization with normal microflora.

Vaginoscopy

The vagina and cervix should be examined with a sterile vaginascope (Fig. 2.7).

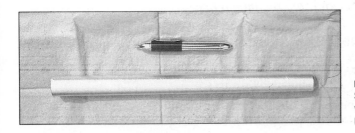

Fig. 2.7
Sterile disposable vaginascope with penlight torch.

Stage of oestrous cycle

This can be classified by the state of relaxation, colour and moistness of the cervix—the oestrous cervix being relaxed, pink and moist, the dioestrous cervix being tight, pale and dry. The classification can be compared with the teasing behaviour and information obtained from utero-ovarian examinations.

Vaginitis

Vaginal inflammation/discharge may be a sign of pneumovagina to corrrelate with the results of perineal examinations. Vaginitis may coexist with acute endometritis, to be confirmed by endometrial examinations.

Vaginal injury

Healed lacerations and, or, rectovaginal fistulae may be a sign of previous parturient or coital trauma.

Cervicitis

Cervical inflammation and/or, discharge may be signs of pneumovagina and/or acute endometritis, as an extension of vaginitis.

Cervial injury and, or, incompetence

These may be signs of parturient or coital trauma and are always poor prognostic signs. Surgical repairs should be attempted for lacerations. Methods for inserting retention sutures, for mares with incompetent cervical closure, have been described, but should not be considered unless constant supervision of the pregnancy can be guaranteed.

Cervical adhesions

Where possible, these should be broken down by digital manipulation. Following this the cervical canal should be treated with daily manipulation with the application of antibiotic and hydrocortisone ointment (e.g. Fucidin-H; Leo Laboratories) to discourage adhesion reformation.

Endometrial cytology

Smears made from vaginal discharges, endometrial smears and, or, uterine washings may be examined for cytological evidence of inflammatory responses.

Endometrial smears

If the mare is in oestrus, the simplest and most practical technique is to insert a simple extended swab, via a sterile vaginascope, through the open, oestrous cervix, and rotate against the endometrial epithelium, harvesting cells and uterine luminal fluid/secretions. The smear is then made by carefully rolling the moist swab onto a prepared slide. Smears may be made from the material harvested in the cups of guarded swabs (e.g. Kallajan Industries, Long Beach, California), collected via a vaginascope, or by manual introduction (Fig. 2.8).

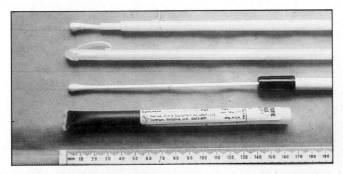

Fig. 2.8 Equipment for collecting endometrial swab and smear samples. (Top) Guarded swab equipment (Kallajan Industries, Long Beach, California) shown in extended and non-extended state. (Bottom) Simple non-guarded swab extended on a sterile extension rod with accompanying transport medium container.

Endometrial aspirates and washings

Smears can be made from fluid samples aspirated from, or saline washes collected from the uterus via Foley-type egg-flushing catheters (Sherwood Medical, St Louis, Missouri), or insemination pipettes (Fig. 2.9).

Smear preparation

A variety of fixation and staining methods give satisfactory results. Experience suggests that Romanowsky-type pre-stained slides (Testsimplets; Boehringer Mannheim GmbH) provide very practical and good quality smears, simply and rapidly, with minimal equipment, using the following techniques (Fig. 2.10):

(1)   Make the smear by rolling (like paint onto a wall) to minimize artefacts, into the pre-stained area. Label with the name of the mare, date, etc. (Fig. 2.10A).
(2)   Incubate on the bench at room temperature for two to three minutes.
(3)   Wash off the background stain under a gently running cold water tap (Fig. 2.10B).
(4)   Allow the smear to dry and then coverslip.
(5)   Panchromatic staining results are obtained as for all Romanowsky-type stains (Fig. 2.10C).

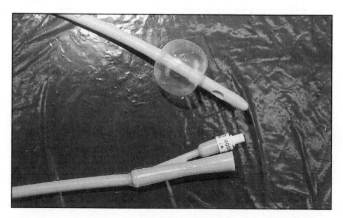

Fig. 2.9
Proximal and distal ends of a Foley-type egg-flushing catheter (Sherwood Medical, St Louis, Missouri) with bulb inflated.

(A)

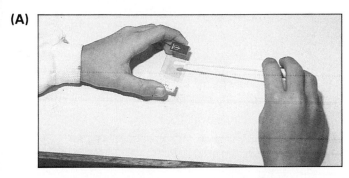

(B)

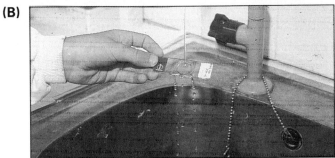

(C)

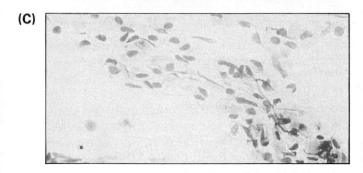

Fig. 2.10
Smear preparation.

Interpretation

The presence of endometrial epithelial cells is used as a measure of smear quality, indicating a diagnostically interpretable endometrial sample, whereas the presence of vaginal epithelial cells (Fig. 2.11) indicates an unsatisfactory vaginal/cervical sample.

The presence of leucocytes (Fig. 2.12) indicates an inflammatory response. Polymorphonuclear leucocytes (PMNs) indicate

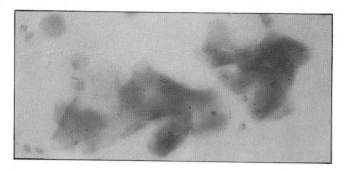

Fig. 2.11
Vaginal epithelial
cells.

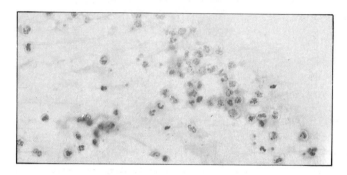

Fig. 2.12
Leucocytes.

acute inflammation and, or, infection, i.e. acute endometritis.
For purposes of comparative reporting, numbers of PMNs are
designated as: −, none seen; + −, <0.5%; 1 +, 0.5%–5%;
2 +, 5%–30%; 3 +, >30%.

Toxic and degenerative leucocyte changes may be seen in
severe acute endometritis. The presence of lymphocytes is
unusual, but may indicate chronic inflammation. Endometrial
smears are not reliable for the diagnosis or investigation of
chronic endometritis, for which biopsy techniques should be
used. Erythrocytes and indefinable debris are often seen in
smears taken at "foal heat". Bacteria and fungi, with leucocytes
demonstrating active phagocytosis, may be demonstrated by
Gram/PAS stains (Fig. 2.13).

Experience has shown that in a genitally healthy mare, no
PMNs should be seen in an oestral smear. Less than 1 per
cent may be acceptable in "foal heat" and maiden (1st oestrus
of the season) mares. In older, subfertile mares, <1 per cent
PMNs may warn of local uterine immune incompetence,
indicating the need for prophylactic mating programmes.

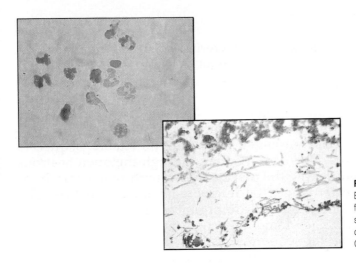

Fig. 2.13
Bacteria (left) and fungi (below) in smears may be demonstrated by Gram/PAS stains.

Endometrial bacteriology

Vaginal discharges, endometrial swabs, uterine washings and endometrial biopsy samples may be examined by bacterial growth. When used concurrently with endometrial smear or biopsy examinations, bacterial endometritis may be diagnosed with confidence.

Endometrial swabs

If the mare is in oestrus, a swab is inserted, via a sterile vaginascope, through the open, oestrous cervix, and rotated against the endometrial epithelium, harvesting cells and uterine luminal fluid and/or secretions. Swabs should be placed immediately into Amies charcoal transport medium and transported to a laboratory, experienced in performing these examinations, as soon as possible and within five days of sampling.

Swabs are routinely plated onto both blood and MacConkey's agar for 48 hours aerobic culture at 37°C and onto chocolated (haemolysed) blood agar, with and without added streptomycin, for six days microaerophilic culture at 37°C.

Interpretation

The clinical significance of bacterial isolates is not made on the grounds of identification alone. Assuming good collection and handling techniques, most bacteria are opportunist pathogens and so clinical features (e.g. cervical inflammation or discharge) and endometrial smear or biopsy results are essential bases for interpretation.

Transient acute endometritis is an inevitable sequel to coitus in mares. Ejaculation occurs through the open oestrous cervix, contaminating the uterine lumen with semen, environmental and external genital microorganisms and debris. The normal, genitally healthy mare produces an efficient transient post-coital acute endometritis, which resolves in 48 to 72 hours, leaving the endometrium in a satisfactory state to receive the fertilized ovum from the fallopian tube at about five days post ovulation. Individual mares with genital abnormality, e.g. pneumovagina, vulval, recto-vaginal or cervical injury, or mares that have impaired local endometrial defence mechanisms, produce a persistent acute endometritis, which invariably results in conception failure or early embryonic loss. Mares with persistent acute endometritis are treated with intrauterine antimicrobial medication, and when appropriate, are treated before and, or, after coitus with a variety of prophylactic techniques.

In 1977 an epidemic endometritis was first recognized which was associated with bacteria which could be seen on Gram-stained smears but could not be cultured using standard aerobic conditions. Microaerophilic culture methods, using haemolysed (chocolated) blood agar, revealed the organism to be a formerly unknown Gram-negative coccobacillus, now named *Taylorella equigenitalis*. Some strains of *K. pneumoniae* and *P. aeruginosa* can cause epidemic endometritis, but in most bacterial (most commonly *Strep. zooepidemicus*, *E. coli*, *Staph. aureus* and *Bacteroides fragilis*) and fungal infections, individual predisposing factors are an essential prerequisite.

Thus the term venereal is used, in the context of equine reproduction, to differentiate bacteria capable of causing epidemic endometritis, involving a stallion and his mares, who may have previously healthy or compromised genitalia, from bacteria which may cause sporadic endometritis, involving individual mares who have compromised genitalia. In

venereal endometritis a common bacterial infection is involved
and only *T. equigenitalis, P. aeruginosa* and *K. pneumoniae* have
so far been shown to have the potential to behave in this
manner. In sporadic endometritis, any of the many aerobic,
microaerophilic and anaerobic bacteria that have been isolated
from the equine genital environment may be involved, in
pure or more commonly mixed culture. As a first step to aid
interpretation, isolates may be broadly classified as follows:

Potential venereal disease bacteria.   T. equigenitalis produces
pin-point, colourless colonies after three days microaerophilic
culture (Fig. 2.14). It is a Gram-negative coccobacillus which
is oxidase and catalase positive. Both the streptomycin
sensitive and insensitive strains are capable of causing
epidemic venereal disease in mares. This organism has not
been isolated in the UK for several years but appears to be
endemic in the non-thoroughbred population of mainland
Europe and therefore routine screening must be maintained.
Treatment with intrauterine penicillin irrigation is usually
successful. The clitoral fossa and sinuses must also be treated
as described above.

  P. aeruginosa produces a luxuriant growth of greenish,
mucoid colonies, with a typically unpleasant smell, usually
overnight under aerobic culture (Fig. 2.15). Occasionally a
typical growth may take 48 hours. Most strains fluoresce in
ultra-violet light. Serotyping may be performed but there is
no known association with venereal pathogenicity.

  Treatment with intrauterine amikacin or ticarcillin and
clavulanic acid (Timentin; Beecham, 3.2 g intrauterine daily)
irrigation may be successful. The clitoral fossa and sinuses
must also be treated as described above.

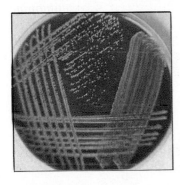

Fig. 2.14
T. equigenitalis culture.

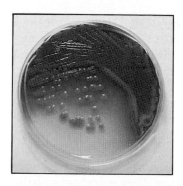

Fig. 2.15
P. aeruginosa culture.

K. pneumoniae produces a luxuriant growth of wet/mucoid colonies overnight under aerobic culture (Fig. 2.16). The colonies are bright pink in colour on MacConkey's agar. Capsule typing, using immunofluorescence or counter-current immunoelectrophoresis may be performed after purification and subculture on Worfel-Ferguson agar. Capsule types 1, 2 and 5 have been associated with epidemic venereal disease in mares but capsule types 7 and 68 have not. Treatment with intrauterine amikacin or gentamicin irrigation may be successful. The clitoral fossa and sinuses must also be treated as described above.

Potential non-venereal acute endometritis bacteria. The following aerobic bacteria are most commonly isolated, in pure or mixed culture, from cases of non-venereal acute endometritis:

Streptococcus zooepidemicus—beta haemolytic
Escherichia coli—haemolytic
Staphylococcus aureus—coagulase positive

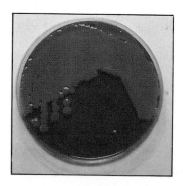

Fig. 2.16
K. pneumoniae culture.

Pseudomonas aeruginosa—"non-venereal" strains
Klebsiella pneumoniae—capsule types 7, 68
Pseudomonas fluorescens
Klebsiella oxytoca
Enterobacter aerogenes
Proteus species

Treatment with intrauterine antibiotic irrigations is indicated where there is concurrent cytological evidence of acute endometritis (see above). These organisms are opportunist pathogens and thus predisposing factors such as pneumovagina or cervical injury and, or, incompetence must also be treated. The choice of antibiotic preparation may be based upon *in vitro* sensitivity tests, but mixed infections with multiple species of aerobes and anaerobes (see below) are common and thus a broad spectrum approach is usually appropriate. Particular care should be taken to avoid insoluble or irritant preparations and, or, vehicles, which are likely to induce chronic endometritis, sometimes encouraging *P. aeruginosa* or fungal superinfection. A 100 ml water soluble mixture of 5 mega units crystalline benzyl penicillin (Crystapen; Pitman-Moore), 1 g neomycin, 40 000 units polymyxin B and 600 mg furaltadone (Utrin wash; Univet), daily for three to five days has been found to be particularly useful as a non-irritant, no-residue, "first choice" approach.

Where there are additional signs of uterine fluid accumulation or pyometra, large volume (5 litres, repeated) intrauterine saline irrigation, with added hydrogen peroxide (2 to 3 per cent), may be used before starting antibiotic treatment. Irrigation may be performed via a Foley-type egg-flushing catheter.

Where there are no demonstrable physical predisposing factors, and a history of recurrent acute endometritis suggests a local immune defect, *in vitro* and *in vivo* research suggests that intrauterine homologous plasma irrigations (a source of complement, important in the opsonization process) may be useful. Blood is collected, from the mare, into a 450 ml evacuated sterile blood collection unit (Travenol). After allowing settlement following centrifugation, the plasma is aspirated into 150 ml evacuated sterile transfer pack units (Travenol) and either used immediately or stored overnight at $+4°$ C. Complement is relatively labile and for longer storage, $-70°$ C conditions are required. Prior treatment with large volume saline flush and, or, antibiotic irrigation is recommended, followed by four to five daily intrauterine irrigations with 150 ml homologous plasma.

Contaminant and/or commensal bacteria.   The following aerobic bacteria are seldom isolated, in pure culture, from cases of non-venereal acute endometritis: *Staphylococcus albus; Streptococcus faecalis; Escherichia coli*—non-haemolytic; *Corynebacterium* species; *Anthracoides* species. Where they are isolated in cases of acute endometritis, treatment should be provided as described above.

Anaerobic bacteria.   Anaerobic culture can be performed using simple anaerobic jars with proprietary sachet systems (e.g. Gas generating kit; Oxoid). Detailed anaerobic culture and identification may, in some cases, require more specialized facilities.

The equine uterus may harbour obligate anaerobes as surface commensals. These organisms normally inhabit the external genital surfaces of mares and stallions and are periodically introduced into the uterus at coitus or in association with genital pathology, e.g. pneumovagina or vagino/cervical injury. They may act as opportunist pathogens where there is epithelial damage, e.g. during the post-partum involutionary period. Synergism with aerobic bacteria may result in mixed infection and active endometritis, possibly, as in other species, by inhibiting uterine leucocyte phago-cytosis, via competition for opsonins. The most common anaerobic isolates from endometrial specimens are: *Bacteroides fragilis; Peptococcus* species; *Peptostreptococcus* species; *Clostridium perfringens; Clostridium sporogenes; Clostridium paraperfringens; Fusobacterium mortiferum; Fusibacter* species.

In the mare, the ubiquitous uterine anaerobe is *B. fragilis*. This species is predominantly penicillin and aminoglycoside resistant, a feature which is pertinent when intrauterine antimicrobial therapy for endometritis is considered. Detailed anaerobic diagnoses are unavoidably time consuming and as mixed infections are common, an antibiotic mixture which contains furaltadone or metronidazole should be used (see above). Failure to do this may account for some cases of aerobe negative persistent endometritis.

Endometrial mycology

Fungal cultures can be performed on Sabouraud's agar. Isolates are sometimes made on simple blood agar plates during aerobic bacterial screening. They are opportunist pathogens and interpretation of significance depends on clinical, cytological and, or, histopathological criteria. The most commonly isolated fungal organisms are: *Candida* and *Mucor* species and *Allescheria boydii*.

Treatment is with intrauterine irrigation with large volumes of saline solution and 2 per cent organic (povidone) iodine.

Endometrial mycoplasmas/ureoplasmas/chlamydia

There is no evidence available as yet to suggest that these organisms have a significant role to play in equine endometritis.

Endometrial virology

There is no evidence available as yet to suggest that viruses have a significant role to play in equine endometritis.

RECTAL PALPATION/ULTRASOUND ECHOGRAPHY

Uterus

During oestrus and anoestrus, the uterus has minimal palpable tone. Diffuse hypoechogenic endometrial oedema delineates the endometrial folds during early oestrus. During dioestrus, the normal uterus should have uniformly palpable tone and no palpable enlargements.

Ventral dilatations are areas of fold atrophy and myometrial stretching which may contain hypoechoic *luminal fluid accumulations* (Fig. 2.17) or large *lymphatic cysts* (Figs 2.18–2.20) which protrude into the uterine lumen, or *lymphatic lacunae* which

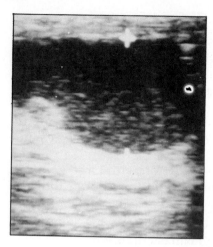

Fig. 2.17
Hypoechoic luminal fluid accumulation (5 MHz linear array ultrasound echographic examination) in the uterus of a mare with a palpable uterine ventral dilation.

occur in the stroma (see later). Both are lined by endothelial cells and contain lymph. Cysts and lacunae are common in multiparous mares over 14 years old and, unless very large and widespread throughout the uterus appear to have no specific effect on fertility. They may be unilocular or multilocular and contain lymphatic fluid.

Pneumouterus may be palpated and confirmed by the demonstration of very hyperechoic bright intraluminal areas (Fig. 2.21). Air may be aspirated into the uterus of mares with

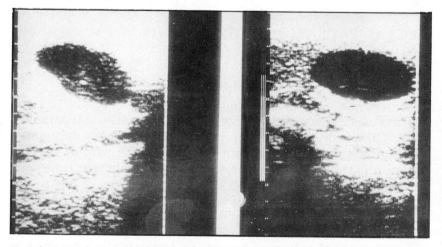

Fig. 2.18 Hypoechoic endometrial lymphatic cysts (3.5 MHz linear array ultrasound echographic examination).

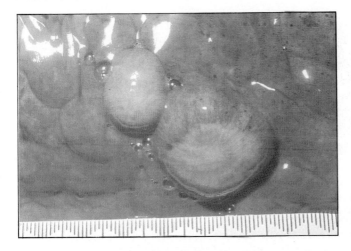

Fig. 2.19
Necropsy specimen, endometrial lymphatic cysts.

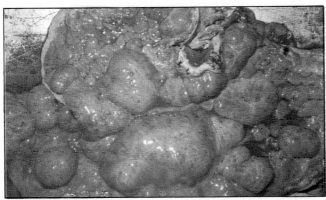

Fig. 2.20
Necropsy specimen, multiple endometrial lymphatic cysts in the uterus of an aged mare with a history of repeated pregnancy failure.

pneumovagina and is a sign that vulval/perineal surgery is indicated (see earlier text).

Pyometra presents as a uniformly enlarged uterus, palpably distended or "doughy", containing hypoechoic fluid, often containing many small hyperechoic particles (Fig. 2.22), giving a "scintillating" echographic appearance. Cases may have cervical adhesions, which may prevent uterine drainage, and these must be identified and treated (see earlier text) if possible. Initial drainage and then saline and hydrogen peroxide flushing may be performed via a double stomach tube system, one placed in a uterine horn (ingress) and the other just inside the internal cervical os (egress). Following this, a course of intrauterine antibiotic and then homologous

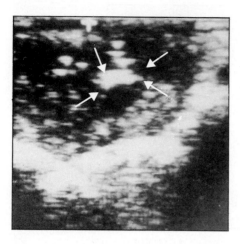

Fig. 2.21
Hyperechoic air (arrowed) (5 MHz linear array ultrasound echographic examination) in the uterus of a mare with pneumouterus.

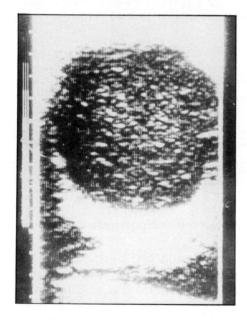

Fig. 2.22
Hyperechoic particles in hypoechoic fluid (3.5 MHz linear array ultrasound echographic examination) in a mare with pyometra.

plasma irrigations (see earlier text) is recommended. The prognosis is always poor for mares with pyometra, but some successes have been achieved since homologous plasma treatment has been used. For intractable cases, suitable for riding, ovariohysterectomy may be indicated.

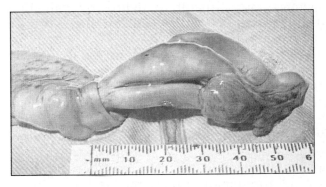

Fig. 2.23
Markedly small ovary.

Ovaries

Palpable follicular activity can be correlated with stage of oestrous cycle and ultrasound echographic examinations can confirm hyperechoic follicles and can reveal hyperechoic corpora lutea.

Markedly small (Fig. 2.23) or absent ovaries, in barren maiden mares suggests *gonadal dysgenesis*. True *cystic ovarian disease*, as seen in some other species, is uncommon in mares. Follicular size is very variable and many large "cysts" appear to ovulate normally. Multifollicular ovaries (Fig. 2.24), perhaps with *ovulation fossa inclusion cysts*, may produce erratic cyclic behaviour and may respond to large doses of exogenous GnRH and then PGF$_{2\alpha}$.

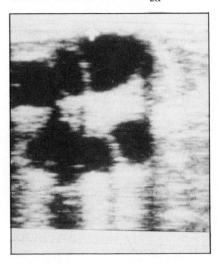

Fig. 2.24
Multifollicular ovary (5 MHz linear array ultrasound echographic examination).

Ovarian *haematomas* are difficult to define by palpation alone, but can be accurately diagnosed by their diffuse hyperechoic appearance (Fig. 2.25).

Granulosa cell tumour is the most commonly diagnosed ovarian neoplasm. The affected ovary is enlarged (Fig. 2.26), palpably hard and the ovulation fossa is not readily palpable. It is echographically polycystic, the cyst walls being relatively thick (Fig. 2.27). The contralateral ovary is small and inactive. The mare may show nymphomania, virilism or maternal behaviour depending upon neoplastic steroidogenesis.

Teratomas may contain teeth or hair. The treatment for these benign granulosa cell tumours and teratomas is ovariectomy.

Adenocarcinomas are aggressively malignant and invariably require euthanasia. Peritoneal fluid analysis may aid diagnosis if exfoliated neoplastic cells are demonstrable.

Fallopian tubes

Palpable or echographic abnormalities of the fallopian tubes are uncommon. *Para-ovarian cysts* or other local developmental abnormalities may be incidental findings. They seldom have a specific effect on fertility.

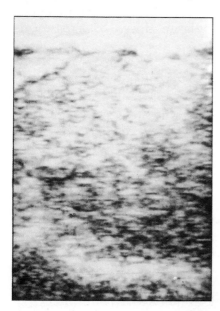

Fig. 2.25
Hyperechoic ovarian haematoma (5 MHz linear array ultrasound echographic examination).

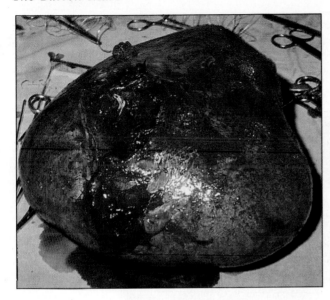

Fig. 2.26
Ovary with granulosa cell tumour.

Extrauterine abnormalities

Organizing *broad ligament haematomas* or *pelvic adhesions* may be detected.

VAGINO/CERVICAL PALPATION

Digital exploration of the cervical canal may reveal lacerations, fibrosis and, or, luminal adhesions. Lacerations may sometimes be repaired surgically and adhesions may sometimes be treated by digital breakdown and the repeated application of antibiotic and hydrocortisone ointment (see earlier text).

ENDOMETRIAL BIOPSY

Basket-jawed (approx. 2 × 0.5 cm) forceps (Fig. 2.28) (55 cm long) (Rocket of London) are essential to provide interpretable biopsy specimens. Non-pregnancy must be confirmed prior to biopsy. One biopsy taken from a mid-horn region is diagnostically representative unless there are palpable uterine abnormalities, where more than one sample should be taken. A mid-dioestral biopsy is recommended as a routine.

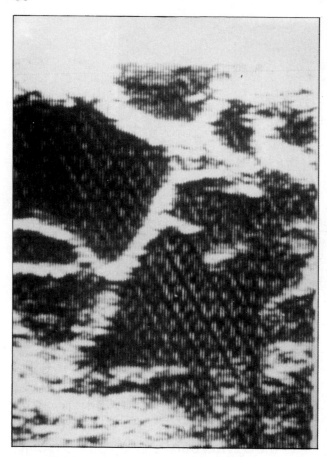

Fig. 2.27
Typical thick hyperechoic walled, hypoechoic polycystic appearance of an ovarian granulosa cell tumour (3.5 MHz linear array ultrasound echographic examination).

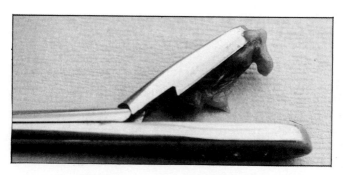

Fig. 2.28
Basket-jawed forceps.

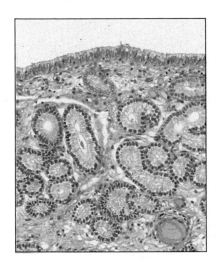

Fig. 2.29
Endometrial biopsy sample, normal oestrus (H&E, × 20 objective).

Cyclic histology

During oestrus the luminal and glandular epithelial cells become tall columnar (Fig. 2.29) and the apical cytoplasm contains maximal quantities of acid and neutral mucopolysaccharides. Alkaline phosphatase staining is maximal. During dioestrus (Fig. 2.30) the luminal and glandular epithelial cells become low columnar (Fig. 2.31) and the apical cytoplasm contains minimal quantities of mucopolysaccharides and alkaline phosphatase staining is minimal. Acid phosphatase staining is maximal. During anoestrus luminal and glandular epithelial cells are cuboidal (Fig. 2.32) and are histochemically inactive. During early oestrus the glands become straight and stromal oedema is minimal. During anoestrus, the gland

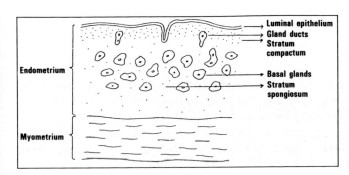

Fig. 2.30
Diagram of the histological architecture of the endometrium of the normal dioestrous mare.

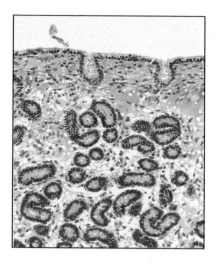

Fig. 2.31
Endometrial biopsy sample, normal dioestrus (H&E, ×
20 objective).

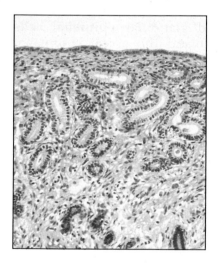

Fig. 2.32
Endometrial biopsy sample, normal anoestrus (H&E, ×
20 objective).

lumens are tightly closed around "impacted" eosinophilic
secretion. Using histological and histochemical criteria (Fig.
2.33), the endometrium can be dated as early oestrus, mid-
oestrus, post ovulation, mid-dioestrus or anoestrus. The
presence of large dioestral ovarian follicles can cause some
confusion.

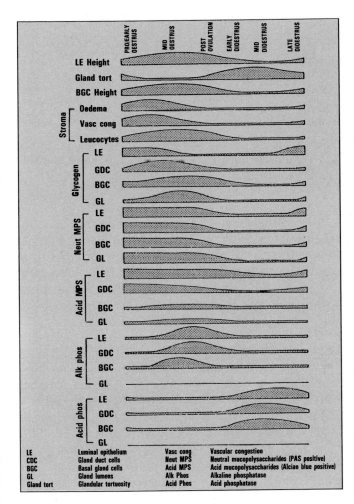

Fig. 2.33
Dating the equine
endometrium using
histological and
histochemical criteria.

LE	Luminal epithelium	Vasc cong	Vascular congestion
CDC	Gland duct cells	Neut MPS	Neutral mucopolysaccharides (PAS positive)
BGC	Basal gland cells	Acid MPS	Acid mucopolysaccharides (Alcian blue positive)
GL	Gland lumens	Alk Phos	Alkaline phosphatase
Gland tort	Glandular tortuosity	Acid Phos	Acid phosphatase

Histopathology

Mixed pathology is common, but specific changes should be
classified and their significance assessed in terms of degree.

Acute endometritis (Figs 2.34–2.36)

Polymorphonuclear leucocytes are seen in the stratum com-
pactum and migrating between luminal epithelial cells.

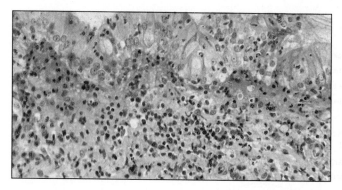

Fig. 2.34
Endometrial biopsy
sample, acute
endometritis, PMN
infiltration of the
degenerate luminal
epithelium and
superficial stroma
(H&E, × 40
objective).

Luminal epithelial degenerative changes may be seen. Eosinophils may be seen in mares with pneumovagina, delayed post-partum involution or following intrauterine medication.

Acute endometritis indicates an inflammatory response, most commonly associated with bacterial infection. Treatments are as described earlier.

Chronic infiltrative endometritis (Fig. 2.37)

Mononuclear cells, i.e. histiocytes/lymphocytes and plasma cells are seen diffusely and, or, in focal stromal aggregations.

The presence of these cells indicates a local immune response and therefore previous or on-going antigenic challenge. This may be a healthy sign and therefore no specific treatment is indicated for this lesion alone.

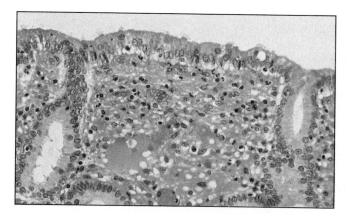

Fig. 2.35
Endometrial biopsy
sample, acute post-
parturient
endometritis,
eosinophil infiltration
of the stroma (H&E,
× 40 objective).

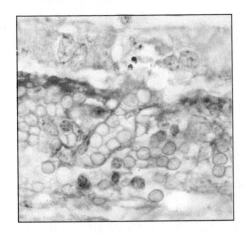

Fig. 2.36

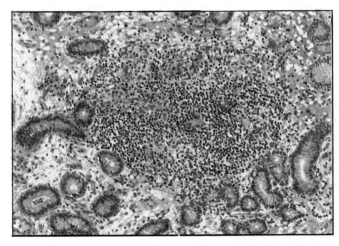

Fig. 2.37
Endometrial biopsy
sample, focal
Infiltrative
endometritis, diffuse
mononuclear cell
infiltration of the
superficial stroma,
including plasma
cells (H&E, × 40
objective).

Chronic degenerative endometritis

Degenerative changes are seen in the form of gland "nests" (Fig. 2.38), surrounded by lamellae of fibrous tissue, or less commonly, gland "cysts" (Fig. 2.39), lined by epithelial cells. Periglandular, perivascular, or less commonly, diffuse stromal fibrosis is seen (Fig. 2.40). Pools of tissue fluid may be seen scattered in the stroma. Lymphatic "lacunae", lined by endothelial cells and containing lymph, may be seen in the stroma (Fig. 2.41). It is unusual to sample a lymphatic cyst (Fig. 2.42) using biopsy techniques, but these are thought to have a similar pathogenesis.

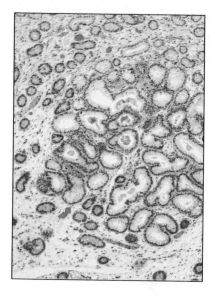

Fig. 2.38
Endometrial biopsy sample, chronic degenerative
change, gland "nest" (H&E, × 10 objective).

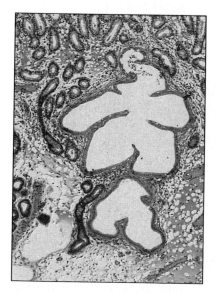

Fig. 2.39
Endometrial biopsy sample, chronic degenerative
change, gland cysts (H&E, × 10 objective).

These changes indicate chronic endometrial degenerative
disease. This is a progressive condition associated with ageing,
the repeated stimulatory challenges of semen, microorganisms,
external genital and environmental debris, fetoplacental antigens, and the repeated physical challenges of pregnancy,

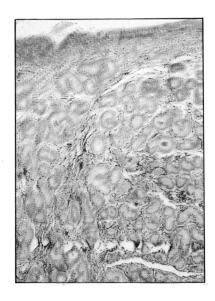

Fig. 2.40
Endometrial biopsy sample, chronic degenerative
change, diffuse stromal fibrosis (Wiegert & Van Gieson,
× 10 objective).

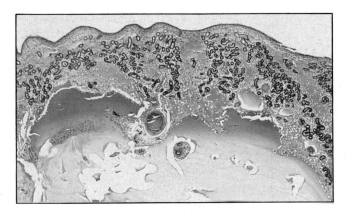

Fig. 2.41
Endometrial biopsy
sample, chronic
degenerative change,
lymphatic lacunae
(H&E, × 4 objective).

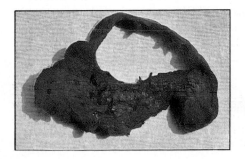

Fig. 2.42
Endometrial necropsy sample, single
endometrial lymphatic cyst, fixed in Bouin's
fluid.

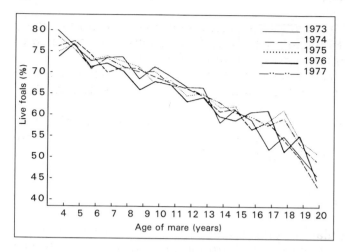

Fig. 2.43
Graph showing the linear decline in fertility potential with age in the thoroughbred mare population of UK and Eire (Jeffcott and others 1982, diagram from Rossdale and Ricketts 1980).

parturition and involution. These changes may, to a large extent, account for the linear decline in fertility with age which has been reported in the thoroughbred mare population (Fig. 2.43) and they are frequently seen in mares who suffer repeated pregnancy failure or prolonged gestation with fetal dysmaturity. Degenerative changes are inevitable to a degree and thus each biopsy specimen must be assessed in terms of the mare's age and parity. Where the degree of degenerative change is considered excessive, treatment with mechanical endometrial curretage (Fig. 2.44) may be attempted. This technique is a method of providing relatively minimal local physical stimulation, with less risk of producing transluminal adhesions than with more aggressive and less controllable chemical "curettage" methods. Improvements in histopathological appearance and fertility can be expected in 50 per cent of mares under the age of 17 years.

   In some cases, recurrent acute endometritis/pyometritis appears to produce diffuse stromal fibrosis, possibly associated with recurrent premature luteolysis and hyperoestrogenism.

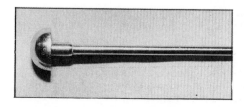

Fig. 2.44
Distal end of instrument suitable for mechanical endometrial curettage in mares.

Successful treatment of the acute endometritis, followed by normal dioestrous periods and then pregnancy, can sometimes reduce the signs of diffuse stromal fibrosis.

Treatment with intrauterine "hot" (50°C) hypertonic saline has been suggested for mares with excessive tissue fluid accumulation or lymphatic lacuna formation.

Where there is concurrent acute endometritis, dimethyl sulphoxide (1 per cent) may be added to the antibiotic mixture in an attempt to aid stromal penetration.

Endometrial atrophy

Diffuse glandular atrophy is seen following prolonged ovarian inactivity and is therefore a normal temporary feature during winter anoestrus.

True endometrial atrophy (Fig. 2.45), with luminal and glandular atrophy, may be seen in aged mares, usually in association with senile ovarian malfunction. Rarely, it has been seen in younger mares following severe recurrent acute endometritis with *Pseudomonas aeruginosa* infection. No treatment is successful and retirement should be recommended.

Endometrial hypoplasia (Fig. 2.46)

Diffuse glandular underdevelopment has been seen in barren maiden mares, sometimes in association with ovarian cyclic irregularities. It appears to be a feature of relative genital

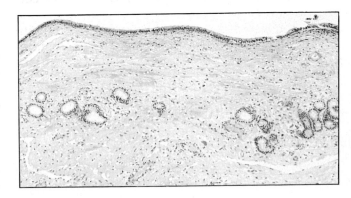

Fig. 2.45
True endometrial atrophy.

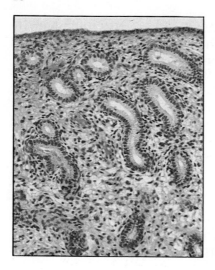

Fig. 2.46
Endometrial hypoplasia.

immaturity and usually resolves, without treatment, in time. Where the degree of hypoplasia is marked and the ovaries are abnormally small, or where the condition persists, the possibility of gonadal dysgenesis should be considered.

Endometrial hyperplasia (Fig. 2.47)

Diffuse glandular hyperplasia with hypersecretion is a normal feature of the post-partum or post-pregnancy failure period.

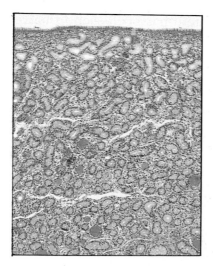

Fig. 2.47
Endometrial hyperplasia.

Normal glandular architecture and secretory activity is usually achieved by 10 to 12 days but occasionally may persist for weeks, if not months, when it is considered pathological. Concurrent acute endometritis is frequently seen. Treatment with 50 iu oxytocin in 500 ml saline by intravenous drip has been used with good results.

In some cases, recurrent acute endometritis/pyometritis appears to produce diffuse glandular hyperplasia, possibly associated with recurrent premature luteolysis and hyperoestrogenism. Successful treatment of the acute endometritis will reduce the signs of diffuse glandular hyperplasia.

HYSTEROSCOPY

Examinations may be made with the fibreoptic endoscope or video endoscope (Fig. 2.48). The latter instrument has a more powerful light source and this gives better visualization.

Lymphatic cysts, luminal fluid accumulations, transluminal adhesions and endometrial neoplasms may be studied. Biopsy specimens obtained with instruments supplied for passage through the endoscope are too small to be diagnostically useful, but conventional biopsy forceps may be used alongside the endoscope, under direct visualization. Attempts to remove large lymphatic cysts and possibly tumours may be made, via the endoscope, by puncture or wire thermocautery.

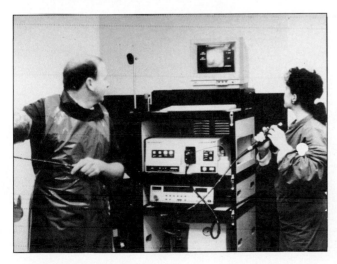

Fig. 2.48
Video endoscope.
(Photo courtesy of Dr
W. R. Allen, Equine
Fertility Unit,
Newmarket.)

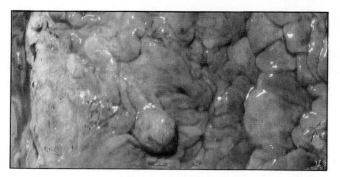

Fig. 2.49
Leiomyoma/fibroleiomyoma.

Endometrial neoplasia

Leiomyoma/fibroleiomyoma (Fig. 2.49) is the most commonly diagnosed equine uterine tumour. They are usually small and benign, and have no primary effect on fertility. Treatment, by surgical removal, is only indicated where the tumour is large, when it may be pedunculated, and may cause persistent endometrial haemorrhage and secondary endometritis.

One case of malignant *adenocarcinoma* (Fig. 2.50) has been recorded in the literature. The mare had respiratory signs and necropsy examination confirmed pulmonary metastases.

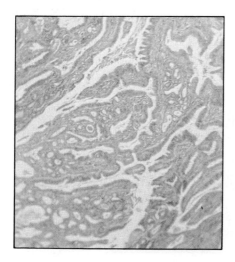

Fig. 2.50
Endometrial adenocarcinoma (H&E, × 4 objective). (Slide kindly supplied by Dr D. Gunson, University of Pennsylvania.)

LAPAROSCOPY

This technique has been used to study the physiology of ovulation in mares and might be helpful in the investigation of ovarian abnormality.

FALLOPIAN TUBE PATENCY TEST

A starch grain periovarian injection and vaginal retrieval test has been described. Necropsy studies suggest that blockage of the fallopian tubes is very rare in mares, and bilateral blockage primarily resulting in infertility has not been reported.

CHROMOSOME ANALYSIS

Leucocytes may be harvested from buffy coat cultures from heparinized jugular blood samples, taken under sterile conditions, and karyotype analysis may be performed after specialized processing.

LAPAROTOMY

Rarely, midline or flank laparotomy may be indicated for the investigation and, or, treatment of uterine or ovarian abnormality.

PROGNOSIS

Following detailed investigation, diagnoses are made and treatments are performed. Prognoses should be given in two stages:

(1) after the first complete diagnostic evaluation; and
(2) after treatment and follow-up examinations, assessing the ability of the mare to respond to treatment and, or, compensate for the abnormalities diagnosed. Failure to respond to specific treatment clearly confers a poor prognosis.

PROPHYLAXIS

After a satisfactory follow-up examination, a prophylactic plan should be formulated, if indicated, particularly in cases with advanced chronic degenerative endometrial disease and, or, with histories of recurrent acute endometritis. The aim should be to reduce endometrial challenge at mating to a minimum and to aid early resolution of inevitable post-coital acute endometritis by use of *minimal contamination techniques*. This can be achieved in populations of horses where registration authorities allow, by the use of artificial insemination with washed and antibiotic-extended semen. Where this approach is not applicable, pre-breeding techniques should be used:

(1)   Satisfactory endometrial swab and smear test results should be obtained at the current oestrous period.
(2)   An apparently normal, on-going, mature ovarian follicle should be palpable.
(3)   Mating should be arranged as close as possible to the estimated time of likely ovulation.
(4)   Pre-breeding semen extender, containing antibiotics, should be instilled into the mare's uterus as soon as possible prior to mating. A suitable extender is as follows: dried, low fat skimmed milk ("Marvel"), 2.5 g; gelatin, 0.5 g; glucose, 5.0 g; penicillin (crystalline), 300 mg; streptomycin (crystalline), 300 mg. This powdered mixture may be stored at +4°C in sealed plastic sachets, prior to use following reconstitution at 37°C in 100 ml sterile water.
(5)   Luteinizing hormone in the form of HCG or GnRH should be used to hasten ovulation.
(6)   150 ml homologous plasma should be instilled into the uterus 24 hours after mating.
(7)   A second mating during that oestrous period should not be allowed.

Pregnancies achieved should be identified as "high risk" and should be monitored by serial ultrasound scan. Unnecessary maternal stress should be avoided throughout pregnancy. Prolonged gestation identifies the fetus as "high risk" and neonatal critical care facilities should be prepared.

CONCLUSIONS

Few mares are truly infertile. With an accurate diagnosis, rational treatment and careful management, many can be encouraged to breed successfully. Management "teamwork" is a vital limiting factor and sufficient commitment is required from the owner, in terms of interest and finance, from the stud farm manager, in terms of interest and staff time and facilities, and from the veterinary surgeon, in terms of interest, time, knowledge, experience and provision of the necessary equipment.

REFERENCES AND FURTHER READING

Asbury, A. C. (1987). *Current Therapy in Equine Medicine,* 2nd edn, (ed. N. E. Robinson), p. 508. Philadelphia, W. B. Saunders.

Baker, C. B. & Kenney, R. M. (1980). *Current Therapy in Theriogenology,* (ed. D. A. Morrow), p. 721. Philadelphia, W. B. Saunders.

Ball, B. A. (1988). *Veterinary Clinics of North America: Equine Practice* **4,** 263.

Blue, M. G. (1987). *Current Therapy in Equine Medicine,* 2nd edn, (ed. N. E. Robinson), p. 511. Philadelphia, W. B. Saunders.

Bowen, J. M. (1987). *Current Therapy in Equine Medicine,* 2nd edn, (ed. N. E. Robinson), p. 567. Philadelphia, W. B. Saunders.

Evans, L. E., Tate, L. P., Cooper, W. L. & Robertson, J. T. (1979). *Proceedings of 25th Annual Convention of American Association of Equine Practitioners,* p. 483.

Frauenfelder, H. (1987). *Current Therapy in Equine Medicine,* 2nd edn, (ed. N. E. Robinson), p. 516. Philadelphia, W. B. Saunders.

Ginther, O. J. (1986). *Ultrasonic Imaging and Reproductive Events in the Mare.* Equiservices, Cross Plains, Wisconsin.

Greenhof, G. R. & Kenney, R. M. (1975). *Journal of the American Veterinary Medical Association* **167,** 449.

Jeffcott, L. B., Rossdale, P. D., Freestone, J., Frank, C. J. & Towers-Clark, P. F. (1982). *Equine Veterinary Journal* **14,** 185.

Kenney, R. M. (1978). *Journal of the American Veterinary Medical Association* **172,** 241.

Kenney, R. M., Bergman, R. V., Cooper, W. L. & Morse, G. W. (1975). *Proceedings of the 21st Annual Convention of the American Association of Equine Practitioners,* p. 327.

Kenney, R. M. & Ganjam, V. K. (1975). *Journal of Reproduction and Fertility* Suppl. 23, 335.

Liu, I. K. M. (1987). *Current Therapy in Equine Medicine,* 2nd edn, (ed. N. E. Robinson), p. 500. Philadelphia, W. B. Saunders.

Liu, I. K. M. (1988). *Veterinary Clinics of North America: Equine Practice* **4,** 221.

Mackintosh, M. E. (1981). *Veterinary Record* **108,** 52.
Pouret, E. J. M. (1982). *Equine Veterinary Journal* **14,** 249.
Powell, D. G. (1980). *Current Therapy in Theriogenology,* (ed. D. A. Morrow), p. 779. Philadelphia, W. B. Saunders.
Ricketts, S. W. (1975). *Equine Veterinary Journal* **7,** 102.
Ricketts, S. W. (1978). Histological and histopathological studies on the endometrium of the mare. Fellowship Thesis, RCVS, London.
Ricketts, S. W. (1981). *Veterinary Record* **108,** 46.
Ricketts, S. W. (1985). *Equine Veterinary Journal* **17,** 3.
Ricketts, S. W. (1985). *Equine Veterinary Journal* **17,** 324.
Ricketts, S. W. (1987). *Current Therapy in Equine Medicine,* 2nd edn, (ed. N. E. Robinson), p. 503. Philadelphia, W. B. Saunders.
Ricketts, S. W. (1987). *Current Therapy in Equine Medicine,* 2nd edn, (ed. N. E. Robinson), p. 518. Philadelphia, W. B. Saunders.
Ricketts, S. W. (1987). *In Practice* **9,** 117.
Ricketts, S. W. & Curnow, E. W. M. (1988). *In Practice* **10,** 204.
Ricketts, S. W. & Mackintosh, M. E. (1987). *Journal of Reproduction and Fertility,* Suppl. 35, 343.
Rossdale, P. D. & Ricketts, S. W. (1980). *Equine Studfarm Medicine,* 2nd edn, p. 1. London, Bailliere Tindall.
Roszel, J. F. & Freeman, K. P. (1988). *Veterinary Clinics of North America: Equine Practice* **4,** 247.
Simpson, D. (1987). *Current Therapy in Equine Medicine,* 2nd edn, (ed. N. E. Robinson), p. 513. Philadelphia, W. B. Saunders.
Van Camp, S. D. (1988). *Veterinary Clinics of North America: Equine Practice* **4,** 229.
Wingfield Digby, N. J. (1978). *Equine Veterinary Journal* **10,** 167.
Wingfield Digby, N. J. & Ricketts, S. W. (1982). *Journal of Reproduction and Fertility* Suppl. 32, 181.

CHAPTER 3

Care of Neonatal Foals— Normal and Abnormal

DAVID R. ELLIS

INTRODUCTION

Good management of the foaling and post-partum environment are important to the health of the neonatal foal but they will be of little help if the foal does not acquire a good passive immunity via colostrum. If a mare is to foal away from home, at a stallion stud for example, it is preferable that she should be moved there about three weeks before her due date so that she can become accustomed to her new surroundings and, in particular, develop immunity to the microflora of that environment which she can pass on to her foal in the colostrum. She should also be given influenza and tetanus vaccine boosters three to four weeks before foaling.

There may be a greater risk of infectious disease at a stallion stud where the population can originate from many different areas or countries—rhinopneumonitis virus abortion is particularly feared. Unfortunately Pneumabort K (Fort Dodge) vaccination does not always prevent virus abortion but it may limit the extent of an outbreak. In advising an owner whether to foal a mare at home, which could be safer from infectious disease, the veterinary surgeon must consider carefully whether the owner's experience, staff and facilities present a greater risk to the viability of the foal and the health of the mare. If the potential value of a foal is large, the foaling might be better delegated to more experienced hands in spite of the risk of infection.

The passive immunity which the newborn foal should receive in the colostrum is jeopardized if the mare runs milk during the days or weeks before foaling. Premature lactation is usually initiated by early separation of the placenta close to the cervical pole which may result from placentitis or twin pregnancy and can pre-empt abortion. In many cases the cause of the early separation is unknown and a healthy foal is born. Unfortunately early placental separation and consequent premature lactation are irreversible and the loss of immunoglobulins and colostrum renders the foal very susceptible to infectious disease. Therefore, donor colostrum which is collected from other foaling mares after their foals' first feeds, stored deep frozen, and thawed slowly but not microwaved, is given (300 to 400 ml) either by bottle or stomach tube for the first feeds. If the foal has already sucked, the large molecules in colostrum will still be absorbed for up to six hours afterwards. If colostrum is not available, broad spectrum antibiotic cover can be given by injection for three to four days, or plasma can be given intravenously.

Plasma can be harvested by collecting up to 4 litres of blood from the mare into acid citrate dextrose and after centrifugation or letting it stand for a few hours the plasma is drawn off and given immediately or stored deep frozen for future use. Provided it is given slowly and the pulse rate is monitored, 1 litre can safely be given intravenously to young foals. If desired a second litre can be given two days later.

The young foal's immune status can be measured using a zinc sulphate turbidity test on its serum or CITE Foal IgG Test Kit (Iddex) on blood collected in EDTA. To avoid false results the foal should be at least 18 hours old and a level of less than 4 mg/litre indicates that treatment with plasma or antibiotics would be wise. Tetanus antitoxin should also be given a day or two after birth if the IgG is low or the mare unvaccinated. Similar tests can be used on the mare's or donor colostrum to check its antibody level prior to feeding.

FOALING AND THE FIRST HOURS

Foaling should be supervised quietly and calmly with only necessary interference being made, such as checking the foal's presentation, episiotomy if the vulva has had Caslick's surgery, traction if the second stage is unduly prolonged and supporting the foal if it is delivered with the mare standing. Delivery usually occurs in recumbency and afterwards the mare and foal should be left to rest. The umbilical cord ceases pulsation after a few minutes and then separates or can be parted at the weak point, 3 to 5 cm external to the abdomen. Ideally, blood loss is minimal, ligation is unnecessary and the umbilical stump can be powdered or sprayed with antibiotic. Caustic applications such as iodine are not recommended as they can blister the adjacent skin.

The normal foal quickly rights itself on to its brisket and may start sucking or chewing movements. Shivering is normal and initially the respiratory rate may be rapid (80 per minute) and pulse rate about 100 per minute. These parameters gradually settle to approximately 40 and 80, respectively, during the first few hours. Attempts to stand are made within minutes and on average a normal foal will stand within two hours and suck within four hours of birth.

Some foals, for no obvious veterinary reason, are less competent than others and may need careful support and guidance. Sucking should be observed carefully to ensure that the foal sucks the teat and swallows milk; some foals suck everywhere but the teat and if attendants are deceived and stop supervision it could be some hours before this is realized, by which time the foal may have become weak and need artificial feeding. A newborn foal should not be left more than six hours without a feed.

The normal foal dries off quickly and can maintain a normal body temperature of approximately 38°C soon after birth even in a wide range of ambient temperatures. The clinician will judge a foal's thermoregulation not only with a thermometer but by observing its coat, behaviour and the temperature of the distal limbs, which should always feel warm. The ability to maintain body warmth is an important sign of health during the neonatal period.

Soon after its first feeds the foal may stale and pass meconium but, even in normal foals, these functions can be delayed for some hours. In the early days staling, which often occurs after feeding, is a good indicator that a foal is taking sufficient milk. On many stud farms the foal's passage of meconium is encouraged by the routine administration of an enema when the foal is a few hours old. The foal is restrained standing and the enema is given gently via a soft rubber tube using either 150 ml liquid paraffin or up to 1 litre of warm soapy water. Proprietary human enemas (Fletcher's Phosphate; Pharmax) are also effective. Meconium is usually expelled soon afterwards but if the soft yellow dung is not apparent for a few more hours and straining continues then the enema is repeated.

For ease of management foals are best handled and guided with the mare from the early hours onwards. After a few days a head collar can be put on and they are led with the mare. From the first day they are best allowed into a paddock which ideally should be small, and the mare and foal should have it to themselves for a few days to get accustomed to each other and the larger space before mixing with others. It has been known for mares to swap foals in the first day or two after foaling without rejection. Presumably maternal ties to the foal take some days to develop and this is also seen in first foaling mares which seem to reject or can even savage their foals in the early days. Such mares may need to be held to allow the foal to suck and extreme cases may need muzzling. A twitch or sedation is rarely necessary. Another important reason for not allowing newborn foals out into large paddocks with other mares and foals is that when first freed, some mares gallop excessively and their foal can become exhausted and injure itself trying to keep up. It is in this way that fracture of the proximal sesamoid bones, the commonest fracture in young thoroughbred foals, is caused.

A first foaler, or occasionally an older mare, may fail to provide sufficient milk for her foal. An early sign is restlessness in the foal which repeatedly goes to the udder and sucks for short periods but does not stale or lie down and rest afterwards. Over a day or two it becomes apparent that the foal has hollow flanks and is not thriving. This may be a temporary problem, particularly in first foalers, and milk production gradually improves with demand. Occasionally a mare will not let milk down and this can be detected and aided by the intravenous injection of 2 to 4 iu of oxytocin in water. If present, milk will be let down immediately. There is no specific treatment for agalactia in mares so one has to rely on regular demand for milk and feeding the mare cut grass *ab libitum*. The foal can be supplemented with milk products such as Aintree Foalmilk (Day, Son & Hewitt), Horsepower (Volac) or Equilac (Pegasus, Eire, Gilmer & Brown) using a bottle or bowl. If the foal refuses, then periodic supplementary feeds (two or three times daily) may be given by stomach tube, but the foal must not be discouraged from sucking the mare as this is the best stimulus to lactation. The older foal (from a week or so) may eat milk pellets from a creep manger. It is rare that fostering is necessary bcause of a mare's failure to accept her foal or produce milk. Persistence is usually rewarded.

CARE OF THE NEONATAL FOAL IN ILLNESS

When the clinician first attends the neonatal (less than four days old) foal showing signs of illness, he has a limited list of differential diagnoses. Generally he will have to treat the foal empirically and institute good nursing until further tests or clinical observation give a definite diagnosis and consequent treatment.

NURSING THE RECUMBENT FOAL

(1) Ensure a clean, dry, deep bed with a rug, towel, or blanket under the foal's head to protect its eyes.
(2) If in lateral recumbency the foal should be turned at least once an hour to prevent hypostatic congestion of the lower lung.
(3) Maintain a good ambient temperature (21°C may be necessary) in the stable, but allow adequate ventilation.
(4) If the foal is comatose, shocked, dehydrated or the limbs feel cold, bandage them with gamgeee or cotton wool from feet to knees and hocks, and cover body with a rug or jersey.

FEEDING THE NEONATAL FOAL (Fig. 3.1)

(1)   The foal should be fed every two to four hours, or hourly if practicable

(2)   If there is no suck reflex, small volumes (up to 300 ml) should be given at body temperature by stomach tube with the foal held standing or supported in sternal recumbency. Take great care with the deeply comatose foal which may die during feeding, presumably due to circulatory collapse—the attendants may get the wrong impression that you have drowned it!

(3)   An indwelling stomach tube of narrow bore (0.8 cm diameter) can be inserted to thoracic oesophageal level and sutured to the lateral canthus of the nostril. It can be severed at the nostril or left long and attached to a head collar but between feeds this end should always be corked to prevent ingestion of air. In some foals this latter complication and the consequent colic makes the indwelling tube impractical. Another concern arising from the use of the long term indwelling stomach tube is the development of gastric ulcers.

(4)   During the recovery phase, particularly in dehydrated cases, a foal may learn to feed from a bowl (Fig. 3.2) before it can suck a bottle or the mare. This can be very beneficial to the foal and veterinary surgeon but, as with bottle feeding, great care must be taken not to wean the foal from the mare to the attendants. Electrolytes, dextrose and Ovigest (Coopers Pitman-Moore) or Lectade (Beecham) can be given in place of milk, particularly if the foal has had diarrhoea.

(5)   When a foal recovers its suck reflex, particularly after convulsive disorders, it may need some guidance to feed from

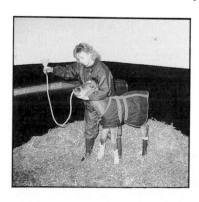

Fig. 3.1
Feeding the neonatal foal by stomach tube. Bandaging distal limbs and fitting a rug help maintain body temperature during neonatal illness.

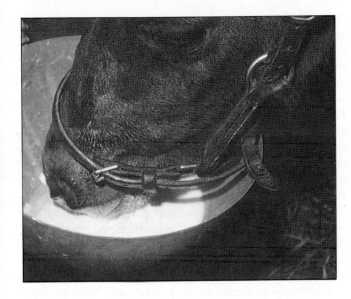

Fig. 3.2
Foals often drink from a bowl if supplementary feeding is required or during recovery from illness, sometimes before the suck reflex returns.

the mare. Leaving the mare unmilked and the foal hungry for a couple of hours beforehand may improve the chances of success.

(6) If the foal is not sucking, the mare must be milked out completely and carefully every 1.5 to 2 hours. This routine is especially important on the second and third days when the milk may suddenly diminish. If this seems to be happening, more frequent milking is necessary. This is the most important step to maintain lactation but feeding the mare fresh cut grass and allowing short periods of exercise may be helpful.

MEDICAL CONSIDERATIONS

(1) If the foal is born in a collapsed or distressed state, oxygen can be administered via a nasal tube or mask. It has been shown that its peak effect is achieved after two minutes and further administration thereafter does not significantly increase blood oxygen levels.

(2) Whenever possible, good quality colostrum should be the foal's first feed as discussed above. Feeding alone can have a rapid beneficial effect on weak and mildly convulsive foals.

(3)   Even if a good passive immunity is acquired, the recumbent foal should be given antibiotic cover. Unless a specific organism is isolated from the placenta, the foal's blood or joints and sensitivity tests indicate otherwise ampicillin and neomycin are preferred, administered twice or three times daily.

(4)   Dehydration or prolonged recumbency often result in entropion and this is best corrected using two vertical mattress sutures to make a tuck in and evert the lower eyelid.

(5)   Constipation is a common complication of prolonged artificial feeding and is treated by adding 50 ml of liquid paraffin to a feed once or twice daily.

(6)   Frequency and volume of urination give a rough guide to the adequacy of feed intake and fluid balance, except of course in the foal with a patent or ruptured bladder. However, serial blood analysis will give a reliable indication of dehydration and progress during treatment.

(7)   Bedsores, if already present or acquired, are best treated with calamine lotion, better bedding and more frequent turning (see Fig. 3.4).

(8)   Indwelling vascular catheters can be inserted for sampling and treatment and, if kept carefully and changed every 24 to 36 hours, reduce the risk of phlebitis and running out of patent veins after a few days.

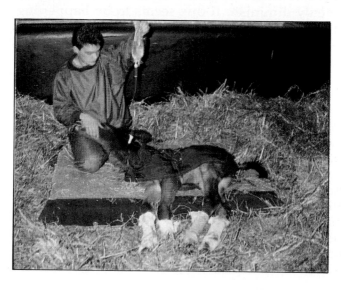

Fig. 3.3
Intravenous fluid therapy is crucial to the recovery of foals which collapse with neonatal septicaemia or diarrhoea and dehydration. The soft rug prevents straw abrading the eye while the foal is recumbent.

(9)   Fluid therapy is crucial to the recovery of foals which collapse with neonatal septicaemia or diarrhoea and dehydration (Fig. 3.3). Lactated Ringer's or Hartmann's solution alternated with dextrose saline can be given intravenously up to 3 litres at a time. Early in the recovery phase electrolytes can be given by mouth if the foal will drink from a bottle or bowl.

(10)   Anticonvulsant therapy is the one treatment that few experienced clinicians are dogmatic about. Many drugs have been tried and some which may theoretically be contraindicated such as acetylpromazine or detomidine which dramatically reduce blood pressure, have been very successful in some instances. Primidone (2 to 3 g initial dose for a 50 kg foal) has a good safety record but has the disadvantage of having to be given by stomach tube and taking up to 20 minutes to have its effect—that is a very long time if the foal is convulsing badly. However, it is ideal for maintenance of anticonvulsant effect. Diazepam (0.1 mg/kg) or phenytoin (5 mg/kg) can be given intravenously to effect.

DISEASES/DISORDERS SEEN IN THE NEONATAL PERIOD

RHINOPNEUMONITIS VIRUS

If a foal is born in a collapsed or extremely weak state the first disease to rule out is rhinopneumonitis virus (EHV1) abortion. Although rare, such cases can be born at term and may be jaundiced. A blood sample from the newborn foal which has a total leucocyte count of less than $1 \times 10^9/l$ is strongly suggestive of EHV1 infection. Even the best nursing and medical care is unlikely to be successful and urgent steps must be taken to reduce spread of the infection to other mares, particularly if they have 10 or more days to reach term. Experience shows that following a primary abortion, foals born within 10 days are unlikely to be affected. Virology on heparinized blood, nasopharyngeal or placental swabs or a post mortem examination would confirm the diagnosis but may take a few days so hygiene and isolation measures should be taken on clinical suspicion of EHV1.

PLACENTITIS

Foals have similarly been born in a collapsed state from mares with severe bacterial placentitis, for example *Klebsiella pneumoniae*.

PREMATURE FOALS

The premature foal is unlikely to survive if it is born before 300 days of gestation. Causes include placentitis (fungal or bacterial) or twin pregnancy. Those born later than 300 days may progress well even if they need artificial feeding in their early hours.

The danger period for the more premature foal is in the first 24 to 48 hours when they can slip relentlessly downhill and die. Such cases show typical signs of being grossly undersize, weak, slow to stand or suck and having a prominent forehead and short soft coat. The tongue may be a bright red colour and the foals chew persistently. The fetlock joints may be flaccidly hyperextended. When born markedly undersize (less than 36 kg for a thoroughbred) foals cannot grow to normal adult size and if the conformation is poor, serious thought must be given before spending great veterinary effort and expense treating them.

FRACTURE OF THE RIBS

Fracture of the ribs is the most common birth injury and it is believed to occur as the foal's keel-like sternum passes through the pelvis simultaneous to the elbows. It occurs particularly when mares foal standing up or get up and down during delivery. They fracture unilaterally in varying numbers between ribs 2 and 10 and close to the costochondral junction. If displacement occurs the pleura, lung, pericardium or even myocardium may be penetrated. In the latter two cases death ensues rapidly but if damage is less extensive the foal may be recumbent or have difficulty in standing. Diagnosis is not difficult in the severe case as the ventral chest is asymmetric. If only two or three ribs are broken signs may be limited to palpable crepitus, oedema or a haematoma. Special care in handling and limitation of exercise are advisable and second-ary complications such as sequestration, abscesses, chronic pleurisy or penetration of the diaphragm are rare.

NEONATAL MALADJUSTMENT SYNDROME
(Fig. 3.4)

Inability or unwillingness to suck may be a feature of foals with fractured ribs but the newborn foal which suddenly

(A)

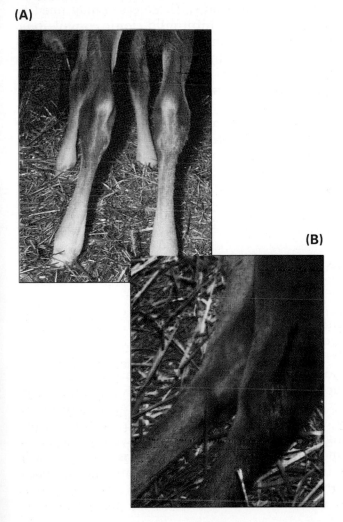

(B)

Fig. 3.4
(A) Mild cases of neonatal maladjustment syndrome which fail to lie down for long periods often develop oedema in the distal limbs. (B) Insufficient bedding often results in bedsores: a typical early example on the lateral side of the hock which can result in local cellulitis or sloughing of skin.

loses or has no suck reflex and which chews on the finger inserted into its mouth is most likely a case of neonatal maladjustment syndrome, originally designated as dummies, wanderers or barkers in ascending order of severity. It occurs at varying times following a normal birth and an early sign may be respiratory distress. Most cases pass meconium rapidly. The mildest case may just lack a suck reflex and require feeding for the hours or days it takes the reflex to develop. The more severely affected foal lacks the suck reflex but is also blind and walks aimlessly round the stable not recognizing the mare or attendants. These cases may need to be laid down to rest and may exhibit mild clonic convulsions. Most severe convulsions are characterized by sweating, forced hyperpnoea, extensor rigidity and opisthotonus. In rare cases expiratory barking or yapping noises are made. Death can occur during severe convulsions.

These cases are a harsh test of medical and, particularly, nursing care. The rate of recovery is variable and may take as long as one or two weeks. Most cases can return to normal and it is very rare for a foal never to learn to suck—the last step in recovery.

SEPTICAEMIA AND PNEUMONIA

The septicaemic foal can be difficult to differentiate from those with severe neonatal maladjustment. It will probably have failed to receive colostrum and at any time in the neonatal period becomes increasingly lethargic, weak and unwilling to suck. Pneumonia, diarrhoea, dehydration or joint distension may also become evident. The total white blood cell count may be below normal but exhibit a shift to the left and toxic changes in the cells. If the foal survives the acute stage, there may be a leucocytosis later in the disease. Pneumonia is likely to occur if the lungs are incompletely expanded as in many foals with neonatal maladjustment syndrome.

DIARRHOEA

Diarrhoea in the neonatal period can lead to rapid dehydration and collapse. A few cases show colicky signs. Rotavirus is diagnosed by virological techniques performed on a faecal sample. These and other serious outbreaks can benefit from prophylactic or therapeutic administration of plasma by stomach tube, after it has been harvested from a mare whose foal has recovered. If a *Salmonella* species is cultured from affected foals, special precautions such as isolation and screening of contacts must be undertaken. Whatever the aetiology and prescribed antibiotics, intensive fluid therapy and maintaining body warmth are the most important facets of treatment.

SEPTIC POLYARTHRITIS

In all cases likely to have an infectious cause, culture of blood or a rectal swab prior to the first empirically chosen treatment can pinpoint the most effective antibiotic. Culture of synovia is often unrewarding but microscopic examination of a Gram-stained smear of sediment may reveal the type of bacteria involved. Septic polyarthritis should always be suspected if a young foal is found lame. Rest, intensive antibiotic treatment and drainage and flushing of infected joints are important. In some neonatal cases the infection spreads to overcome the foal so quickly that even intensive treatment is unavailing.

RETAINED MECONIUM

The most common cause of colic in the neonatal period is retained meconium which impacts in the rectum or occasionally higher in the large bowel so that tympany develops anterior to the obstruction. Signs usually appear at 16 to 24 hours of age and foals continue to suck in spite of persistent straining and intermittent colic. Pain is rarely intense and only if the case is prolonged do they weaken and stop sucking. Digital examination of the rectum reveals firm, dry meconium impacted anterior to the pelvic inlet. With good lubrication and great care pieces can be removed digitally or by using a meconium spoon or canine whelping forceps. However, especially when using instruments contusion, oedema (and even rupture) of the rectal wall may occur. Small doses of flunixin meglumine (50 mg intravenously or intramuscularly) relieve the pain well and enemas should be accompanied by laxatives. Unless removed mechanically, such as with a meconium spoon, the meconium may take more than 24 hours to clear, but surgery is hardly ever necessary. Great care should be taken to ensure that the cause of colic is known before flunixin is given as it could mask the signs of more serious surgical colics.

RUPTURE OF THE BLADDER

Rupture of the bladder is also characterized by persistent straining, but small amounts of urine may be passed. Signs appear at 36 to 48 hours old at the earliest and the foal gradually ceases to suck and weakens while the abdomen enlarges. The rate of deterioration is in direct proportion to the size of hole in the bladder and consequent leakage. With the foal held in lateral recumbency the abdomen is trocarized under local anaesthesia anterior to the navel and just lateral to the midline. As much urine as possible should be drained and surgical repair undertaken one to two hours later. This delay is sensible in order to lower the pressure of urine on the diaphragm, the uraemia and hyperkalaemia, thereby reducing anaesthetic risk. If any intravenous fluids are given they should contain sodium chloride and not any potassium. Some clinicians catheterize the bladder and instil methylene blue dye which is then recovered via the paracentesis to confirm the diagnosis. Pervious urachus does not warrant surgery and usually heals with daily local antiseptic dressing. In rare, but usually older cases, the urachus may leak internally mimicking a ruptured bladder and the entire navel is removed surgically. The navel may also require removal in rare cases with chronic infection or abscessation.

HAEMOLYTIC DISEASE

Foals with haemolytic disease can show clinical signs of anaemia, jaundice, haemoglobinuria, hyperpnoea and fatigue as early as 24 hours of age. If so, the anaemia is peracute and transfusion should be urgent. Severity of haemolysis varies greatly and most cases are diagnosed between two and four days old. Mild cases may show slight anaemia and jaundice and not need treatment. Diagnosis is confirmed by haematology and a direct sensitization test. Giving washed erythrocytes from the dam is simpler than finding a matched donor for an exchange transfusion and is quite effective. Collect 4 to 5 litres of the mare's blood in acid citrate dextrose and have a hospital or large laboratory, such as the Animal Health Trust, centrifuge, wash the cells and resuspend them in isotonic

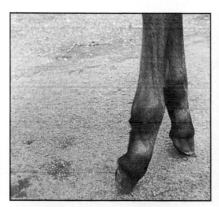
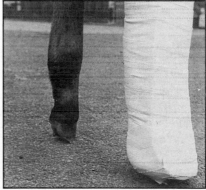
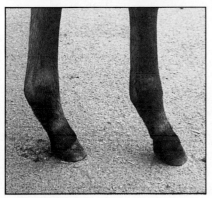

Fig. 3.5
Careful, well padded application of a fibreglass splint to the distal limb for one or two days at a time can allow the foal with flexural deformity (knuckling over) of the fetlock or below to maintain a normal posture by bearing weight on the foot rather than the pastern or fetlock.

saline to yield 2 to 3 litres, which is given intravenously to the foal. Following diagnosis or treatment haemolytic foals should be rested and not overexerted for at least three weeks.

CONGENITAL LIMB DEFORMITIES

Congenital limb deformities require careful assessment before treatment is instituted. Most angulations, hyperextensions and hyperflexions improve spontaneously during the first days of life. If the foal knuckles over, well padded splint support is necessary (Fig. 3.5) and in all cases exercise should be controlled so that the deformed foal does not overtire. Those born with severe carpal contracture may have multiple deformities (e.g. scoliosis, eventration, anencephaly) and require destruction rather than treatment. Immediate surgery is hardly ever necessary for limb deformities in newborn foals.

REFERENCES AND FURTHER READING

In Depth Seminars: B. Neonatal Disease Therapy and Management (1982). *Proceedings of the 28th American Convention of the American Association of Equine Practitioners* **28**, 341.

Koterba, A. M. (1989). *Equine Veterinary Education* **1**, 9.

Neonatal Equine Disease (1985). *Veterinary Clinics of North America: Equine Practice* **1**, No. 1.

Paediatrics (1986). *Proceedings of the 32nd American Convention of the American Association of Equine Practitioners* **32**, 107.

Panel: Management and Treatment of the Premature Foal (1983). *Proceedings of the 29th American Convention of the American Association of Equine Practitioners* **29**, 127.

Panel: Paediatrics (1985). *Proceedings of the 31st American Convention of the American Association of Equine Practitioners* **31**, 127.

Perinatology, *Equine Veterinary Journal* Supplement 5 (1988). (ed. P. D. Rossdale, M. Silver, and R. J. Rose).

Rossdale, P. D. (1972). *Equine Veterinary Journal* **4**, 117.

Rossdale, P. D. & Ricketts, S. W. (1980). *Equine Stud Farm Medicine*, 2nd edn. London, Bailliere Tindall.

CHAPTER 4

Pneumonia in the Foal

TIM MAIR

INTRODUCTION

Infections constitute a major cause of disease and mortality in neonates of all species. It is estimated that approximately 33 per cent of foal deaths occurring within the first two months of life are caused by bacterial infections. The respiratory tract is one of the major portals of entry for bacteria and other pathogens into the body and it is therefore not surprising that pneumonia is one of the most common manifestations of infection in the young foal. Pneumonia is a major cause of economic loss to the horse breeding industry, not only because of fatal infections, but also because of losses associated with growth retardation, decreased work capacity, and expense of treatment.

AETIOLOGY AND PATHOGENESIS (Fig. 4.1)

Infection of the lower respiratory tract may occur alone, or in conjunction with a more generalized infection. In the majority of cases, one or more predisposing factors exist.

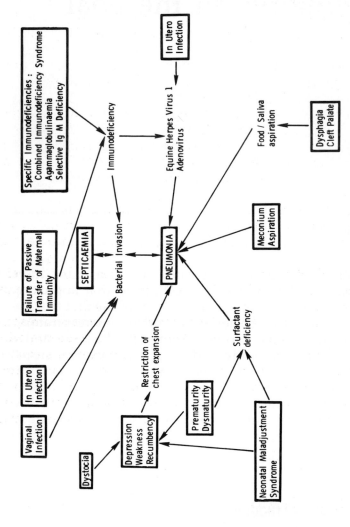

Fig. 4.1 External and internal factors associated with development of pneumonia in the foal.

(1)   Intrauterine infection by bacteria and fungi may result in fetal death caused by placental insufficiency, or infection of the fetus. However, most neonatal infections originate from the vagina or external environment.

(2)   Failure of passive transfer of maternal antibodies is the most common predisposing cause of neonatal infection. Foals which fail to obtain sufficient colostrum are susceptible to infection.

(3)   Other immunodeficiency states (in particular, combined immunodeficiency syndrome of the Arabian breed) also predispose to infection.

(4)   Inadequate quantities of lung surfactant result in atelectasis and increased susceptibility to pneumonia. This may be important in premature foals (born at a gestational age between 300 and 320 days) and dysmature foals (born at a gestational age longer than 320 days but showing signs of prematurity).

(5)   Atelectasis and the presence of hyaline-membrane-like material in the aveolar ducts are frequently present in foals suffering from the neonatal maladjustment syndrome. Such cases are predisposed to the development of pneumonia.

(6)   Recumbency and other conditions which restrict chest expansion result in congestion of the lungs which predisposes to pneumonia.

(7)   The inhalation of foreign material into the lower respiratory tract can result in a chemical bronchopneumonia which rapidly becomes secondarily infected. Aspiration of meconium may occur during birth, especially in cases where there is fetal stress or asphyxia. Aspiration of food and saliva can occur as a result of dysphagia, or structural abnormalities of the upper alimentary or respiratory tracts (such as cleft palate).

CAUSES (Table 4.1)

Bacteria

Bacterial pneumonia is the most common form of lower respiratory tract infection encountered in the young foal. The bacteria most commonly involved are those associated with septicaemia. Mixed bacterial infections are common.

Viruses

Primary viral pneumonia is rarely diagnosed except for equine herpes virus I (rhinopneumonitis). Adenovirus infection is a common complication in combined immunodeficiency syndrome.

Protozoa

Pneumocystis carinii causes interstitial pneumonia in immuno-deficient animals, in particular foals suffering from combined immunodeficiency syndrome.

CLINICAL SIGNS AND DIFFERENTIAL DIAGNOSIS (Table 4.2)

The characteristic signs of pneumonia include: coughing; mucopurulent nasal discharge; tachypnoea and dyspnoea; fever; and depression.

Table 4.1 Major pathogens associated with pneumonia in the foal.

Bacteria	Viruses	Protozoa
Streptococcus zooepidemicus Other *Streptococcus* species *Escherichia coli* *Klebsiella pneumoniae* *Pasteurella multocida* *Actinobacillus* species *Pseudomonas aeruginosa* *Enterobacter* species *Salmonella* species *Bordetella bronchiseptica* *Rhodococcus equi* *Staphylococcus* species	Equine herpes virus I Adenovirus	*Pneumocystis carinii*

Table 4.2 Differential diagnosis of respiratory distress in the newborn foal.

Primary		Secondary
Pulmonary	Non-pulmonary	
Pneumonia	Upper airway obstruction	Persistent fetal
Hyaline membrane	Pleuritis	circulation
disease	Space-occupying lesions	Acute blood loss
Aspiration syndromes		Metabolic acidosis,
Transient tachypnoea		hypoglycaemia
		Cerebral haemorrhage
		and, or, oedema

(1) In septicaemic foals there may be few overt signs indicating pulmonary infection, despite the presence of significant lung pathology. The signs of septicaemia most commonly appear at two days of age and include progressive dullness and lethargy, and a reluctance to suck; subsequently, signs of specific organ dysfunction may become apparent. The first indication of pneumonia in such cases may simply be tachypnoea; this must be differentiated from other causes of respiratory distress.

(2) Pneumonia unassociated with septicaemia (Fig. 4.2) may occur at any age up to six months, but most commonly occurs within the first two months. The clinical signs vary according to the severity of the infection.

(3) *Rhodococcus equi* is an uncommon cause of pneumonia in the UK but it may become endemic on certain farms. The clinical disease may be subacute (sudden onset of severe pneumonia which is rapidly fatal) or chronic (prolonged, unresponsive pneumonia with unthriftiness). The clinical signs often do not become apparent until a large amount of lung damage has occurred.

(4) Perinatal infection with equine herpes virus I (Fig. 4.3) usually presents clinically during the first week of life. The signs include weakness, lethargy, failure to nurse, congestion of the mucous membranes, respiratory distress, tachycardia and a variable body temperature. Diarrhoea develops in some cases.

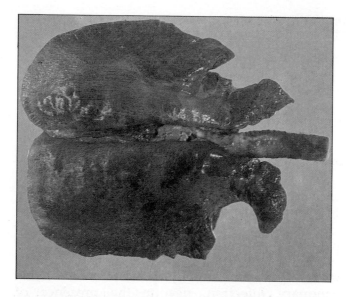

Fig. 4.2
Patchy pulmonary
consolidation
associated with a
mixed bacterial
pneumonia in a four-
month-old
thoroughbred foal.

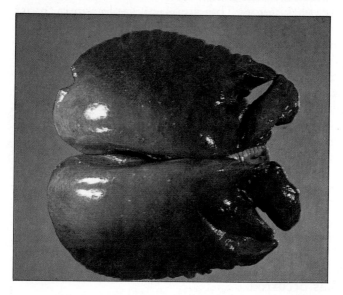

Fig. 4.3
Severe, diffuse
pneumonia in a two-
day-old Arabian foal
associated with
equine herpes virus I
infection.

(5) Adenovirus infection is most frequently recognized in
Arabian foals suffering from combined immunodeficiency
syndrome. The signs of pneumonia occur when protection
derived from colostral antibodies has waned (which may be
from a few days to several months depending on the amount

and quality of colostral transfer). Concurrent infection by a variety of bacteria and *Pneumocystis carinii* is common in such cases.

EVALUATION OF THE FOAL WITH PNEUMONIA (Fig. 4.4)

CLINICAL EXAMINATION

The foal's temperature, pulse rate and character, respiratory rate and character, attitude, exercise tolerance, and appetite should be assessed.

The respiratory rate of the newborn foal is normally high (70 to 80/minute) but decreases to about 30/minute by 12 hours. Normal breathing is quiet, with no flaring of the nostrils or exaggerated thoracic or abdominal movements. The character of any cough or nasal discharge, and the state of hydration should be evaluated.

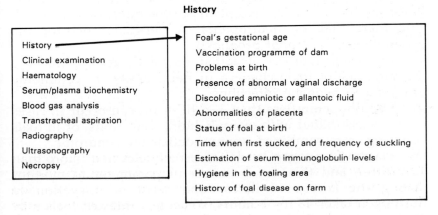

History

History	Foal's gestational age
Clinical examination	Vaccination programme of dam
Haematology	Problems at birth
Serum/plasma biochemistry	Presence of abnormal vaginal discharge
Blood gas analysis	Discoloured amniotic or allantoic fluid
Transtracheal aspiration	Abnormalities of placenta
Radiography	Status of foal at birth
Ultrasonography	Time when first sucked, and frequency of suckling
Necropsy	Estimation of serum immunoglobulin levels
	Hygiene in the foaling area
	History of foal disease on farm

Fig. 4.4 Evaluation of the foal with pneumonia.

The thorax should be thoroughly auscultated. Lung sounds are usually heard more easily in the foal than in adult horses, and inspiratory sounds are louder than expiratory sounds. Loud or harsh lung sounds are suggestive of pneumonia, but it must be remembered that harsh sounds may be present when the respiratory rate is elevated for any cause, even in the absence of pulmonary disease. Crackling and wheezing sounds may both be present in pneumonia, but significant disease can be present without any obvious auscultatory abnormalities; in many cases the lung sounds may appear worse during the recovery stage of the disease. An absence of lung sounds in a certain area is suggestive of consolidation, or the presence of a pulmonary abscess or pleural fluid. Percussion of the thorax is easily achieved in the foal and can aid in the detection of consolidation, abscesses or fluid lines.

The mucous membranes should be assessed for their colour and the capillary refill time. Cyanosis is very rarely detected even when the arterial oxygen tension is dangerously low.

HAEMATOLOGY

Laboratory findings in foals with pneumonia and other infections are variable and depend on the severity and stage of infection.

(1)   Leucocytosis or leucopenia are considered as typical findings in infections, but they are not invariably observed.
(2)   Most foals with bacterial pneumonia show a neutrophilia (at least 10×10^9/litre), except in severe infections in which case there may be neutropenia. A persistent neutropenia generally carries a poor prognosis.
(3)   Increased numbers of immature (band) neutrophils, and the presence of toxic changes in neutrophils are commonly observed in neonatal infections.
(4)   Lymphopenia (less than 1×10^9/litre) can occur in cases of stress associated with overwhelming infections, or in foals suffering from combined immunodeficiency syndrome.
(5)   Plasma fibrinogen levels are usually elevated (more than 4.0 g/litre), and this can be a useful parameter to monitor during the course of illness and recovery. Elevation of fibrinogen takes 48 to 72 hours, so acutely infected foals may process normal fibrinogen levels.

(6) Other haematological parameters can provide useful information especially in foals suffering from concurrent septicaemia. The packed cell volume, haemoglobin concentration and red blood cell numbers all increase in dehydration and, or, shock. However, these parameters decrease during the first 36 hours of life in normal foals, and they may also be reduced in response to chronic infection.

SERUM/PLASMA BIOCHEMISTRY

(1) Serum or plasma protein levels may be monitored to assess the state of hydration. The total protein concentration becomes elevated in dehydration and, or, shock, but the level is highly variable in normal foals (4.0 to 7.0 g/dl in post-suckle serum), so a single measurement is not a reliable indication of the hydration status.
(2) Hypoglycaemia is a common finding in septicaemia, especially in foals younger than 24 hours of age.
(3) Plasma lactate levels become elevated in septic shock due to decreased perfusion of tissues and a shift towards anaerobic metabolism.
(4) Creatinine and urea values are often raised in shock due to inadequate renal perfusion.
(5) Foals with concurrent enteritis may develop severe electrolyte imbalances, including hyponatraemia, hypochloraemia and hypokalaemia.
(6) Immunoglobulin G concentration should be assessed (see overleaf) in cases where failure of passive antibody transfer is suspected. Serum IgG levels of less than 400 mg/dl indicate significant failure of passive transfer of colostrum; ideally the serum IgG level should exceed 800 mg/dl.

BLOOD GAS ANALYSIS

Blood gas analysis is extremely useful in the evaluation of the critically ill foal, but the technology may not be readily available in practice. Arterial samples provide the most valuable information about pulmonary function; the great metatarsal and facial arteries are convenient sites for sampling. Samples should be taken into heparinized syringes, and may be stored several hours on ice prior to analysis.

Transtracheal aspiration (Fig. 4.5)

Transtracheal aspiration is the most useful technique for the collection of lower airway secretions for bacteriological culture; it can also be of value in the diagnosis of viral and protozoal infections. The technique is of most value in the investigation of severe acute cases, or chronic unresponsive pneumonia. Although nasal or nasopharyngeal swabs can be used to diagnose viral infections, contamination by upper respiratory

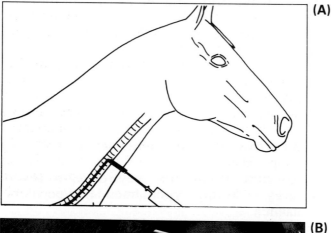

(A)

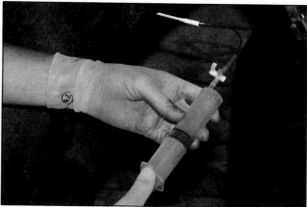

(B)

Fig. 4.5
(A) Diagrammatic representation of the technique of transtracheal aspiration. (B) Transtracheal aspiration in a five-month-old Arabian foal.

tract bacteria precludes their use for the diagnosis of lower airway bacterial infections.

The procedure may be performed with the foal standing or recumbent. Care must be taken to avoid unnecessary stress to the foal and to maintain aseptic technique. An area over the middle third of the cervical trachea is clipped and prepared for aseptic surgery, and a bleb of local anaesthetic is injected subcutaneously over the ventral trachea in the midline. A stab incision is made through the skin, and the subcutaneous tissues are dissected bluntly to the trachea. A variety of needle–catheter combinations may be used to perform the aspiration, but a convenient combination is a 12-gauge, 3 inch over-the-needle catheter with a 5 French gauge canine urinary catheter; for large foals a 10-gauge, 3 inch catheter and an 8 French-gauge urinary catheter can be used. The 12- or 10-gauge catheter is inserted into the tracheal lumen between two cartilage rings, the stylet is removed, and the urinary catheter is passed down into the trachea to the hilar region. Sterile saline (15 to 30 ml) is then infused through the catheter, and immediately retrieved by suction. The flushing and aspiration procedure may be repeated if an adequate sample is not obtained at the first attempt.

The aspirate sample should be submitted for Gram's stain and bacterial culture (including aerobic and anaerobic cultures). Cytological examination may also be useful in determining the type, severity and progression of the lower airway disease; aspirates from animals with pneumonia contain large numbers of neutrophils and degenerative cells (Fig. 4.6).

RADIOGRAPHY (Figs 4.7 and 4.8)

Thoracic radiography can be very helpful in the evaluation of pneumonia in the foal. Radiographs of diagnostic quality can generally be obtained with most portable machines if rare-earth screens are used.

The radiological appearance of pneumonia may give some indication as to the aetiology and pathogenesis of the condition. For example, in cases of aspiration pneumonia, pulmonary consolidation is generally localized to the ventral lung fields. In cases of *Rhodococcus equi* pneumonia, multiple,

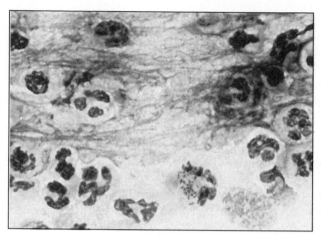

Fig. 4.6
Transtracheal aspiration
from a two-month-old
thoroughbred foal. Gram
stain. There are numerous
polymorphs with strands
of mucus in the
background. There is a
clump of Gram-positive
bacteria in the cytoplasm
of one neutrophil.

ill-defined nodular opacities are often found throughout the lung fields. Frequent sequential radiographs are particularly useful to evaluate therapy and monitor the course of the disease.

ULTRASONOGRAPHY

Ultrasound examination of the thorax can be helpful for the demonstration of pleural fluid or consolidation of peripheral lung tissue. This technique is of greatest value when used in conjunction with radiography.

TREATMENT

SUPPORTIVE CARE

Supportive care is of vital importance in the management of pneumonic foals, especially those with concurrent septicaemia. Such care is often necessary to maintain life until antibiotic therapy and the foal's immune system can control the infection.

(1) Blankets and heat lamps should be used if the foal's temperature falls below 99.0°F.

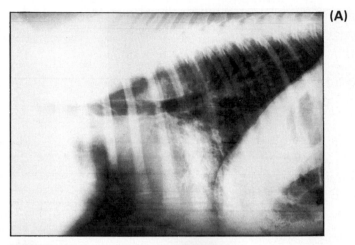

(A)

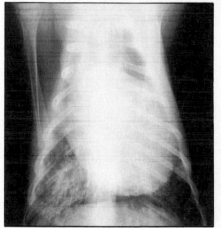

(B)

Fig. 4.7
Inhalation pneumonia in a one-month-old pony foal. The lateral thoracic radiograph (A) shows a fine, reticular infiltrate in the caudal lung, which is intensified ventrally. The ventro-dorsal view (B) shows that the right lung is more severely affected than the left.

(2)   The recumbent foal should be provided with adequate padding and turned frequently.

(3)   If the foal is hypoxic, oxygen (preferably humidified) should be administered (6 to 10 litres/minute) via a face mask or nasal insufflation.

(4)   Intravenous fluids are often necessary in the septicaemic foal to combat cardiovascular collapse. Balanced polyionic fluids, such as lactated Ringer's solution, are usually suitable, and they can be administered at a rate of 30 to 40 ml/kg/hour until adequate volume expansion is achieved. Dextrose saline (5 per cent) may be alternated with the polyionic solution to

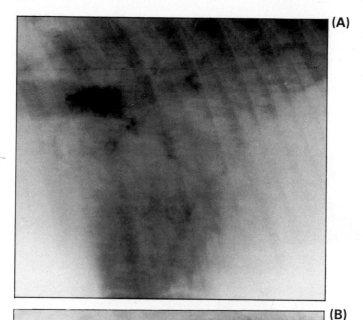

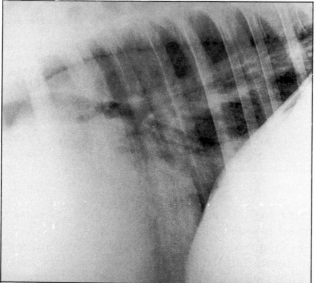

Fig. 4.8
Lateral thoracic radiographs of a 10-week-old thoroughbred foal with bacterial pneumonia. (A) At admission. All lung fields show an increase in opacity, with the greatest consolidation affecting the hilar region. (B) Three weeks later. The lung fields are now virtually normal, although an area of infiltration is still present in the caudal peri-hilar region.

prevent hypoglycaemia. Care must be taken to avoid too vigorous intravenous fluid therapy since foals with pneumonia are susceptible to pulmonary oedema. In mildly dehydrated animals, fluid replacement by the oral or subcutaneous routes may be more convenient.

(5) If hypogammaglobulinaemia (failure of passive transfer) is confirmed, a plasma transfusion is indicated to boost circulating immunoglobulin levels. The dam's plasma is usually suitable, but any donor plasma should first be cross-matched against the foal's erythrocytes. A dose of 20 ml plasma/kg should be administered intravenously (slowly).

ANTIMICROBIAL THERAPY

The rational use of antibiotics depends on the identification of the causative bacteria and their drug sensitivity. However, in many cases treatment must be initiated before the results of culture are available, and in these cases drug selection should be based on an assumption of the most likely bacteria.

The dosages of antibiotics (Table 4.3) necessary for foals are relatively higher than for adults because the extracellular fluid volume in foals is proportionally much higher. However, foals generally require less frequent therapy than adults because of the immaturity of the hepatic microsomal systems. Bactericidal drugs are preferred since many pneumonic foals are immuno-deficient and have an immature reticuloendothelial system.

Streptococcus species are the most common bacteria involved in foal pneumonia, and in most cases, they are susceptible to penicillin. Penicillin G is an excellent first choice for antibacterial therapy; it is bactericidal to most streptococci, has low

Table 4.3 Suggested antimicrobial dosages.

Drug	Route	Dose/kg bodyweight	Times/ day
Amikacin sulphate	im	7 mg	2–3
Amoxycillin, sodium	im	22 mg	4
Ampicillin, sodium	iv im	10–40 mg	4
Chloramphenicol, palmitate	oral	50 mg	4
Chloramphenicol, succinate	iv im	20–25 mg	6
Gentamicin sulphate	iv im	2 mg	2–3
Oxytetracycline	iv	5 mg	2
Penicillin G, procaine	im	20-50 000 units	2
Penicillin G, sodium	iv im	20–50 000 units	4
Trimethoprim-sulphonamide	iv	15–30 mg	2

im intramuscular   iv intravenous

toxicity and is relatively inexpensive. However, since mixed infections are common, and Gram-negative bacteria are commonly involved in septicaemia, broader spectrum cover is usually required. A combination of penicillin with an aminoglycoside drug such as amikacin or gentamicin, or with potentiated sulphonamides give good broad spectrum cover. Alternatively, other beta-lactam antibiotics may be used, e.g. ampicillin or amoxycillin. The aminoglycosides, particularly gentamicin, are nephrotoxic, especially in foals with reduced renal function (e.g. dehydration), so monitoring of renal function (sequential urinalysis and serum creatinine levels) is recommended.

Rhodococcus equi pneumonia poses particular problems in terms of treatment since the organism is an intracellular parasite. Therapy with a combination of erythromycin (25 mg/kg three times a day per os) and rifampicin (5 mg/kg twice daily per os) gives the best results.

ANTI-INFLAMMATORY DRUGS

Although corticosteroids can have beneficial effects in septic shock, they cause profound immunosuppression and should be avoided whenever possible. Non-steroidal anti-inflammatory drugs, such as phenylbutazone and flunixin meglumine, may be of value both in limiting the pulmonary inflammatory reaction, as well as reducing the foal's fever and improving its general attitude and appetite. However, these drugs may predispose to gastrointestinal ulceration and can be nephrotoxic in the hypovolaemic foal. For these reasons they should be used with caution.

BRONCHODILATORS AND MUCOLYTICS

Spasm of airway smooth muscle, and accumulation of excessive lower airway secretions play important roles in the pathophysiology of bronchopneumonia. Bronchodilator and mucolytic drugs can be helpful in combating these processes, and seem to make the foal more comfortable. Clenbuterol and etamiphylline are the most commonly used bronchodilators; the former has the added advantage of aiding clearance of lower airway discharges by increasing ciliary activity.

PHYSICAL THERAPY

Coupage (slapping the foal's chest with a cupped hand) is beneficial in loosening adherent airway secretions.

PREVENTION

The single most important factor in preventing the development of foal pneumonia is ensuring adequate passive transfer of immunoglobulins to the newborn foal. After 24 hours of age, colostrum can no longer be absorbed, and neonates with low serum IgG levels must receive an intravenous source. Serum IgG may be readily measured using a latex agglutination test. Foals with a serum IgG level of less than 800 mg/dl are at risk of infection, and should receive plasma therapy (2 to 4 litres over a two to five day period).

REFERENCES AND FURTHER READING

Beech, J. (1986). *The Compendium on Continuing Education for the Practising Veterinarian* **8,** S 284.

Martens, R. J., Ruoff, W. W. & Renshaw, H. W. (1982). *The Compendium on Continuing Education for the Practising Veterinarian* **4,** S 361.

Rossdale, P. D. & Ricketts, S. W. (1980). *Equine Stud Farm Medicine*, 2nd edn. London, Bailliere Tindall.

Kosch, P. C., Koterba, A. M., Coons, T. J. & Webb, A. I. (1984). *Equine Veterinary Journal* **16,** 312.

Webb, A. I., Coons, T. J., Koterba, A. M. & Kosch, P. C. (1984). *Equine Veterinary Journal* **16,** 319.

CHAPTER 5

Dysphagia in the Horse

TIM GREET

INTRODUCTION

Dysphagia is defined as difficulty in, or the inability, to swallow. This definition is occasionally extended to include any problem associated with eating such as quidding or food dropping. These problems of mastication originate in the oral cavity and will not be discussd here. Lesions originating in the pharynx or oesophagus are the usual causes of dysphagia. However, paralytic or obstructive lesions of the stomach or small intestine may produce nasal reflux of ingesta which may be clinically indistinguishable from dysphagia. Such lesions must therefore be included in any list of differential diagnoses as the major presenting sign of dysphagia is the emergence of food material from the nasal passages. This paper is intended to complement a previous paper by this author (Greet 1986).

PRESENTING SIGNS

Typically there is coughing associated with deglutition and nasal return of food material and saliva. However, the severity of these signs is variable and there may be other more obvious features such as cranial or sympathetic nerve damage, epistaxis, or neurological signs associated with the locomotor system. In some cases, particularly if dysphagia is long standing, a foul smelling purulent nasal discharge may indicate that gangrenous aspiration pneumonia has developed.

CAUSES OF DYSPHAGIA

These can be summarized as follows:

(1)   Pharyngeal obstruction: guttural pouch distension with pus, air, blood; retropharyngeal abscess; foreign body (Fig. 5.1); neoplasia; and subepiglottic cyst.
(2)   Pharyngeal paralysis (Figs 5.2 and 5.3): guttural pouch mycosis; and botulism.
(3)   Palatine abnormalities: clefts and other defects; and rostral displacement of the palatopharyngeal arch.
(4)   Oesophageal obstruction: choke; foreign body; diverticulum; congenital achalasia; and grass sickness.

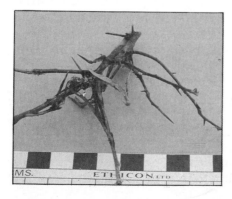

Fig. 5.1
A pharyngeal foreign body from a 13-year-old pony gelding.

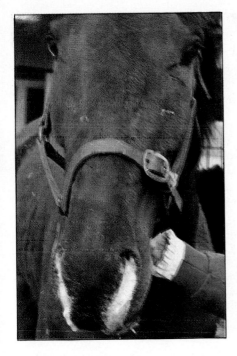

Fig. 5.2
Bilateral nasal discharge of saliva in a four-year-old
thoroughbred mare with pharyngeal paralysis.

EXAMINATION ROUTINE

CLINICAL EXAMINATION

A good history is essential to provide a platform for building
a diagnosis. Occasionally it may provide the only indication
as to the cause of dysphagia.

The horse should be observed carefully to note bodily
condition, character of respiration, head carriage, facial sym-
metry, nasal discharge or evidence of epistaxis. A detailed
clinical evaluation should be carried out, particular attention
being paid to any evidence of aspiration pneumonia (Fig. 5.4)
as this indicates a very poor prognosis. Auscultation of the
chest by stethoscope using a rebreathing bag (Greet 1986) can
be very helpful in this regard to locate adventitious pulmonary
sounds which typically are loudest cranioventrally. Examination of the mouth in cases of botulism may reveal lingual
and masticatory muscle paralysis.

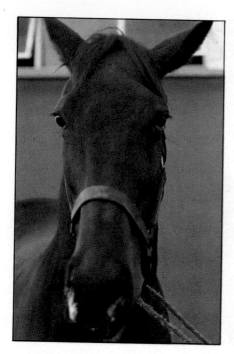

Fig. 5.3
Bilateral nasal discharge because of pharyngeal hemiplegia with left sided facial paralysis in a case of guttural pouch mycosis.

Palpation of the laryngeal and pharyngeal areas will help to identify any swelling or evidence of pain. There may be gross pharyngeal swelling in cases of peripharyngeal haemorrhage, neoplasia or guttural pouch distension. The jugular furrows should also be inspected to check for patency of the jugular veins or the presence of any swelling. Examination should eliminate obvious oral lesions. If neurological signs such as head tilt or ataxia are present, a full neurological investigation must also be performed; although such signs are not commonly associated with dysphagia. The nasal discharge in most dysphagic horses is bilateral although in some cases it may be mainly unilateral (Greet 1986). It usually contains food or saliva and there may be evidence of haemorrhage. The presence of a foetid smell usually indicates severe tissue necrosis as in gangrenous pneumonia but it also occurs with mycosis of guttural pouch.

Eructation is unusual in the horse but is a clinical feature of rostral displacement of the palatopharyngeal arch because of cricopharyngeal muscle aplasia. If nasal reflux of ingesta is

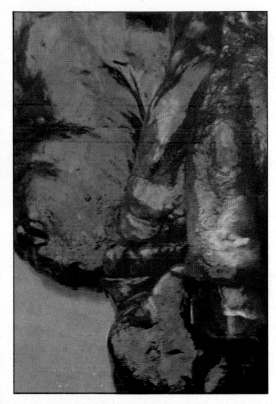

Fig. 5.4
Gangrenous aspiration pneumonia
following pharyngeal paralysis.

associated with a gastric or small intestinal lesion severe
abdominal pain will be a major clinical sign.

ENDOSCOPIC EXAMINATION

A flexible fibreoptic endoscope permits a detailed investigation
of the nasal, pharyngeal, laryngeal and cranial oesophageal
regions. Most causes of dysphagia can be determined accurately using this technique. Palatal defects are readily detected
(Greet 1986) as are most pharyngeal cysts and foreign bodies.
Pharyngeal neoplasia tends to be extensive by the time clinical
signs are apparent and therefore its appearance may be
confused with other conditions such as causes of guttural
pouch distension. The guttural pouches should be inspected
and fungal plaques may be seen easily in most cases of
mycosis (Greet 1986), although in horses with recent epistaxis

the lesion may be obscured by a large haematoma or by fresh haemorrhage. A word of warning here: it is surprisingly easy to disrupt a blood clot in the guttural pouch during endoscopy which may induce an embarrassing or even fatal haemorrhage. It is therefore essential that great care be taken when passing an endoscope into a guttural pouch where there is the suspicion of a mycotic lesion or haemorrhage. Cases of guttural pouch empyema can be recognized by the thick purulent material which exudes from the pharyngeal ostium. However, in some cases there may be no drainage via this route and the affected pouch can be distended markedly causing obvious pharyngeal stenosis. Passage of the endoscope into the pouch reveals thick purulent material and normal anatomical landmarks may be obscured. It should be remarked that some cases of empyema affect both pouches. In guttural pouch tympany guttural pouch distension is frequently marked and sagging of the pharyngeal roof is usually obvious. Insertion of an endoscope into the pouch will deflate it and thus an endoscopic diagnosis is unreliable. Fortunately the condition is very amenable to a radiological diagnosis. Although fracture of the stylohyoid bone is rare, endoscopic confirmation of the lesion in the guttural pouch is possible.

In horses with pharyngeal paralysis the soft palate may be displaced permanently dorsal to the epiglottis. In most horses the paralysis is unilateral usually as a sequel to mycosis of the guttural pouch. Flushing water from the endoscope into the nasopharynx of a healthy horse usually stimulates deglutition, elevation of the soft palate and opening of both guttural pouch flaps. In cases of pharyngeal hemiplegia one side of the pharynx may be obviously immobile during deglutition. In complete paralysis there are no pharyngeal movements and the soft palate remains displaced permanently dorsal to the epiglottis. However, some healthy horses may be reluctant to swallow and it is not uncommon for the soft palate to be displaced dorsally during endoscopy of normal animals. Thus care must be taken before making a diagnosis of complete bilateral pharyngeal paralysis. In cases of pharyngeal paralysis food material is frequently found on the soft palate, particularly around the larynx, and on the floor of the larynx and trachea.

In horses with rostral displacement of the palatopharyngeal arch and cricopharyngeal aplasia (Figs 5.5 and 5.6), the arch

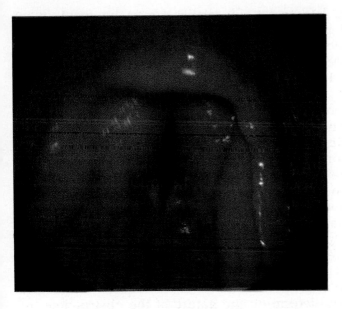

Fig. 5.5
Endoscopic view of
rostral displacement
of the
palatopharyngeal
arch.

is easily seen rostral to the corniculate process of the arytenoid
cartilages. Occasionally the cranial oesophagus may balloon
open permitting a view into its lumen.

Iatrogenic dysphagia may follow the surgical treatment
of laryngeal disease usually by laryngoplasty or partial
arytenoidectomy, because of failure of the protective mechanism of laryngeal closure. In dysphagic horses after the former

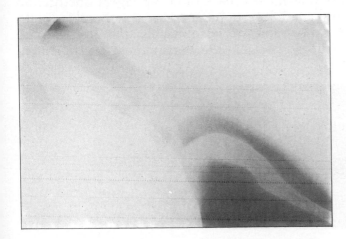

Fig. 5.6
Lateral radiographic
view of horse with
rostral displacement
of palatopharyngeal
arch showing air in
cranial oesophagus
because of
cricopharyngeal
muscle aplasia.

operation the left arytenoid cartilage may be fixed in an overabducted position which can be recognized easily from an endoscopic examination (Fig. 5.7). The postoperative appearance after partial arytenoidectomy can be quite variable. In dysphagic horses the corniculate process may well have been excised.

A flexible endoscope can be passed into the oesophagus, in the same manner as a stomach tube. The best way to examine the oesophagus is by passing the full working length of the endoscope into the horse and inflating the oesophageal lumen with air. Inspect while gradually withdrawing the endoscope. In horses with an obstructive lesion of the oesophagus, food material may be packed cranial to the lesion. Endoscopy may fail to distinguish the precise cause of the problem.

Endoscopic examination after food deprivation of about 24 hours may permit identification of an oesophageal foreign body, usually a twig. Most other cases require radiological investigation to determine the nature of the obstruction.

It must be remembered that an endoscope working length of 2 m or more is usually required for a complete oesophageal inspection of the average horse, pony and even large foals. In the largest horses a 2 m endoscope will not reach the cardia when passed via the nasal passages. If an endoscopic examination of the distal oesophagus is indicated in such animals, an endoscope must be passed via a presternal oesophagotomy.

It is fortunate that most causes of oesophageal obstruction are found in the cranial oesophagus or at the thoracic inlet.

Endoscopic assessment of oesophageal motility can be difficult in the horse because the lumen must be distended

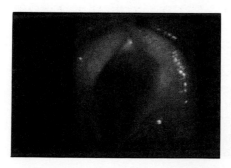

Fig. 5.7
Endoscopic view of hyperabducted left arytenoid cartilage following laryngoplasty treatment of laryngeal hemiplegia. Such cases may show severe dysphagia because of failure of laryngeal protection during deglutition.

with air to allow mucosal inspection. Even in cases of oesophageal incoordination (e.g. grass sickness) prograde oesophageal motility is seen. Conversely it is not uncommon to observe slight intraluminal reflux of fluid while the endoscope is in the oesophagus of normal horses.

RADIOLOGICAL EXAMINATION

In its most sophisticated form radiological evaluation of dysphagia requires expensive equipment beyond the means of most practices. However, it is possible to carry out many useful radiographic investigations of dysphagic horses even using portable or mobile X-ray generators particularly in combination with fast rare earth screen/film combinations.

Plain lateral radiographic views of the pharynx can readily be obtained to demonstrate gross lesions such as a retropharyngeal mass and fracture of the hyoid bone, and guttural pouch empyema or tympany (Fig. 5.8) which can be seen to be compressing the pharynx. Even more subtle lesions such as rostral displacement of the palatopharyngeal arch may be noted and in such cases air may be obvious in the cranial oesophagus because of cricopharyngeal muscle aplasia. A non-focused grid will improve definition and picture quality but may increase exposure factors and more importantly time, precluding its use with lower powered generators. Radiographic examination of the larynx, trachea and cervical oesophagus is well within the range of portable equipment and plain lateral views may be useful to demonstrate some lesions such as a perioesophageal mass or a radio-opaque foreign body.

The oesophagus at the level of the shoulders and thoracic inlet is extremely difficult to investigate and requires the use of high powered equipment and a grid, but views of the thoracic oesophagus may be obtained with portable equipment.

Although plain films may be helpful in dealing with gross lesions particularly in the pharynx, most oesophageal problems or more subtle soft tissue pharyngeal problems require the use of contrast radiography. Oral administration of barium sulphate suspension by syringe (60 ml or more are generally required) followed by at least one swallow, will result

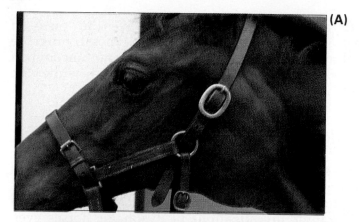

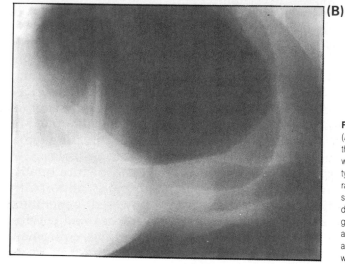

Fig. 5.8
(A) Young thoroughbred foal with guttural pouch tympany. (B) Lateral radiographic view of same foal showing distension of both guttural pouches with air as the foal was affected bilaterally, which is unusual.

in contrast material outlining the oropharynx, lateral food channels and oesophagus (Fig. 5.9). Causes of obstruction such as a subepiglottic mass or oesophageal diverticulum or stricture may be identified easily. In cases of pharyngeal paralysis attempts at deglutition usually produce leakage of barium sulphate into the nasopharynx, larynx and trachea (Fig. 5.10) although some is usually passed into the oesophagus unless there is complete pharyngeal stasis. In foals with soft palatal defects contrast material can usually be seen to have leaked from the oropharynx into the nasopharynx through the defect.

(A)

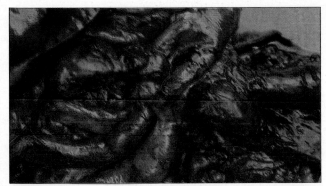

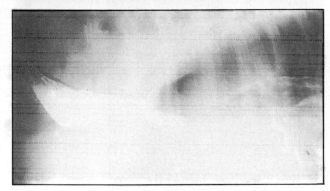

Fig. 5.9
(A) Post mortem examination of thoroughbred foal with a right sided aortic arch. The oesophagus has been obstructed between the right sided aortic arch and the ligamentum arteriosum. (B) Lateral radiographic view of chest of above foal after oral administration of barium sulphate. Note distension of oesophagus cranial to, and marked obstruction to passage of contrast material at the level of, the base of the heart.

(B)

If an obstructive oesophageal lesion is suspected in the mid cervical oesophagus or distally, it may be possible to demonstrate it more satisfactorily by large volume contrast administration. This involves passage of a stomach tube into the most cranial part of the oesophagus administering 100 ml to 1 litre of barium sulphate suspension either neat or with warm water. Serial radiographic views of the oesophagus are then obtained until the site of obstruction is identified. This can be done with a portable generator and fast screen/film combination. In some cases this may demonstrate cases of oesophageal incoordination/dilatation (e.g. in grass sickness) but care must be taken in interpretation as there may be false positives and negatives because the trigger for oesophageal peristalsis is deglutition.

These static radiographic studies can be extremely useful in the investigation of dysphagic horses. However, dynamic investigation using image intensification is a more reliable

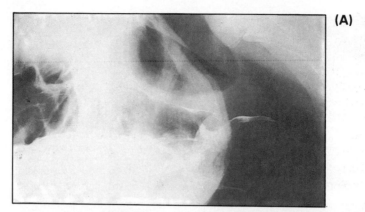

(A)

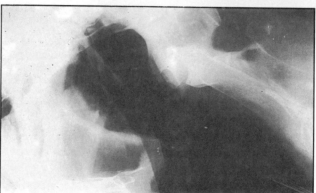

(B)

Fig. 5.10
(A) Lateral radiographic view of horse with pharyngeal hemiplegia after oral administration of barium sulphate. Contrast materal has leaked above soft palate and into larynx. (B) As above with larynx full of contrast material.

and informative technique for evaluating such cases. This procedure is usually allied to oral administration of barium sulphate suspension and permits assessment of deglutition and inspection of the bolus as it passes through the oesophagus to the stomach. This procedure is most informative in cases of pharyngeal paralysis or oesophageal incoordination.

LABORATORY EXAMINATION

Samples of blood collected for routine haematological and biochemical analysis can be used to confirm the presence of infection (e.g. a retropharyngeal abscess or gangrenous pneumonia). In such cases it is common to find elevation of neutrophil counts, fibrinogen and the globulin fraction of the plasma proteins. The recognition of significant anaemia is an important preoperative consideration in cases of guttural pouch mycosis as assessment of blood loss may be difficult (e.g. owner's report may not be reliable).

Bacteriological culture of swabs collected from a nasal discharge, discharging abscess or from a tracheal wash can be used to obtain antibiotic sensitivity and thus appropriate therapy may be instituted.

Collection of fungal material for analysis from plaques in cases of guttural pouch mycosis is not particularly helpful and may precipitate a catastrophic haemorrhage.

Histological examination of a sympathetic ganglion is the only certain method of confirming suspected cases of grass sickness.

DIFFERENTIAL DIAGNOSIS (Table 5.1)

Gangrenous aspiration pneumonia is a possible complication in any horse with dysphagia but other presenting signs may be very valuable in differentiating between causes of dysphagia on clinical grounds.

EPISTAXIS

Pharyngeal and oesophageal foreign bodies may produce scanty epistaxis due to mucosal laceration. More severe epistaxis is usually due to guttural pouch mycosis. These conditions may be readily differentiated endoscopically (Greet 1986).

PHARYNGEAL SWELLING

This is commonly seen in horses with guttural pouch disease when the affected pouch disease is distended by air, pus (Fig. 5.11) or blood. In some cases of guttural pouch mycosis massive peripharyngeal haemorrhage may also contribute to generalized swelling in this region. Another common cause is retropharyngeal abscessation and, much less commonly, pharyngeal neoplasia. These conditions may be distinguished

Table 5.1 Differential diagnosis of dysphagia.

Condition	Other clinical signs	Endoscopy helpful	Radiography helpful Plain	Contrast	Lab helpful
Palatal defect	± Aspiration pneumonia	+ +	±	+	−*
Subepiglottic cyst	Respiratory noise	+ +	±	+	−
Guttural pouch Tympany	Respiratory noise, Marked pharyngeal swelling	+	+ +	±	−
Guttural pouch empyema	Nasal discharge± pharyngeal swelling	+ +	+ +	±	Culture of nasal discharge
Guttural pouch mycosis	Epistaxis, parotid pain, cranial nerve paralysis, ozaena	+ +	±	+	±*
Other causes of pharyngeal paralysis, e.g. botulism	± Aspiration pneumonia, ataxia, recumbency and tongue paralysis in botulism	+	±	+ +	±* Blood test for lead poisoning or botulism
Pharyngeal abscess	Respiratory obstruction, pyrexia	+	+	+	Haematology blood biochemistry culture of nasal discharge
Hyoid bone fracture	± Head tilt, neurological signs	±	+ +	±	−
Pharyngeal foreign body	± Epistaxis, coughing obvious discomfort around throat	+ +	±	±	−

Condition	Clinical signs				Lab test*
Pharyngeal neoplasia	Respiratory obstruction, weight loss	+	+	+	Histology of biopsy
Laryngeal surgery	± Abnormal respiratory noise	++	±	+	−
Rostral displacement of ppa	Abnormal respiratory noise	++	+	±	−
Simple oesophageal impaction	eructation	±	+	++	
Oesophageal stricture	Repeated episodes of dysphagia	±	+	++	
Oesophageal diverticulum	As for stricture	±	+	++	
Oesophageal foreign body		++	±	+	
Grass sickness	Colic, patchy sweating, muscle fasciculation, weight loss	±	−	+	Only post mortem
Megaloesophagus	Young foal	±	−	++	−
Perioesophageal mass	Pyrexia if abscess	+	+	++	Histology of neoplasia haematology/biochemistry if abscess
Gastric impaction, small intestinal obstruction	Severe abdominal pain	±	−	±	±

*Lab test—except culture of tracheal wash if gangrenous pneumonia
ppa Palatopharyngeal arch

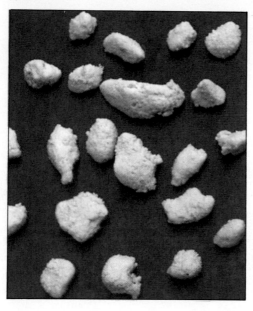

Fig. 5.11
Chondroids from a case of guttural pouch
empyema. These concretions are formed
from inspissated pus.

by endoscopic and radiological examinations and laboratory
tests may also be useful in distinguishing between infection
and neoplasia. However pharyngeal tumours are most satisfactorily investigated by histological examination post mortem
(Fig. 5.12).

RESPIRATORY OBSTRUCTION

Nasopharyngeal compression by an abscess, tumour (Fig.
5.13) or by any cause of guttural pouch distension is the most
usual reason for respiratory obstruction. In some cases
dyspnoea may be so severe that an emergency tracheostomy
is required.

Other less severe causes of respiratory obstruction are the
diseases of laryngeal origin (hemiplegia or chondritis) for
which surgical treatment has induced dysphagia. Pharyngeal
(usually subepiglottic) cysts may produce respiratory obstruction or at least an abnormal respiratory noise. Some of these
horses have concomitant epiglottal entrapment which may
contribute to the noise. Abnormal harsh or "gurgling"
respiratory sounds are often produced by horses with rostral
displacement of the palatopharyngeal arch. This condition is

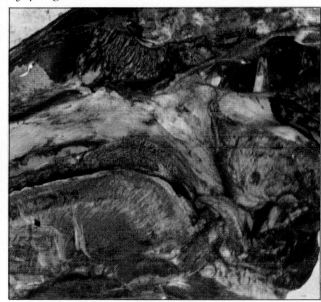

Fig. 5.12
Post mortem
examination of mare
in Fig. 5.13 revealing
large obstructive
pharyngeal tumour
(squamous cell
carcinoma).

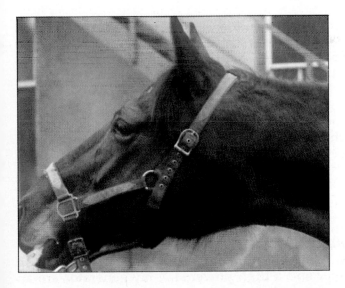

Fig. 5.13
Nine-year-old hunter
mare with severe
dyspnoea and
dysphagia because
of pharyngeal
squamous cell
carcinoma.

quite rare but affected horses usually eructate and can have
low grade dysphagia. Lead poisoning may produce laryngeal
paralysis as well as dysphagia.

NEUROLOGICAL SIGNS

Some cases of guttural pouch mycosis may show severe neurological signs usually because of mycotic damage to the cranial or sympathetic nerves. These include Horner's syndrome, pharyngeal, laryngeal, lingual and facial paralysis. Patch sweating and colic may occur as a result of sympathetic nerve involvement. Cases of grass sickness may show similar signs of sympathetic nerve damage in particular patchy sweating and muscle fasciculation. Any large pharyngeal mass may produce damage to cranial nerves as an effect of pressure but such cases seem very rare.

Botulism may produce profound neurological disturbances which include complete lingual and pharyngeal paralysis, ataxia and recumbency. Lead poisoning has been recorded as a cause of dysphagia but is most commonly seen associated with laryngeal hemiplegia.

ABDOMINAL PAIN

Nasal reflux of food material associated with abdominal pain is usually the result of an obstruction of the cranial gastrointestinal tract, e.g. small intestinal volvulus, intussusception or gastric impaction, and is due to passive reflux (Fig. 5.14). However, in grass sickness the nasal reflux of food material is probably the result of neurological disturbance of oesophageal motility. Rarely, abdominal pain may accompany guttural pouch mycosis and this is thought to be the result of sympathetic nerve damage.

CONCLUSION

The investigation of dysphagia in the horse involves a variety of techniques. Although sophisticated equipment such as an image intensifier and a high powered X-ray generator are an invaluable aid, much diagnostic investigation can be carried out under practice conditions using endoscopy and portable or mobile radiographic equipment. As with any approach to differential diagnosis much information can be obtained from a good history and a thorough clinical examination.

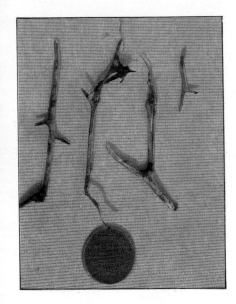

Fig. 5.14
Foreign bodies removed by oesophagostomy from
cranial oesophagus of a two-year-old pony gelding
with severe dysphagia.

Thus even if a case has to be referred for a specific diagnostic procedure the differential diagnostic list can be narrowed considerably prior to referral.

REFERENCE

Greet, T. R. C. (1986). *In Practice* **8**, 49.

CHAPTER 6

Headshaking in Horses

TIM MAIR AND GEOFF LANE

INTRODUCTION

The term "headshaking" is defined as the abnormal condition when a horse shakes its head in the absence of obvious extraneous stimuli, and with such frequency and violence that it becomes difficult or dangerous to ride, or appears to be distressed.

Headshaking is one of the most poorly understood conditions which affects the riding horse and is a cause of great frustration to both owners and veterinary surgeons alike. Obviously, an ability to move the head quickly and to shake it in a rotary manner should be considered a normal behavioural feature that forms part of the defence mechanism of the species, to avoid, for example, harassment by biting flies. This same type of behaviour is sometimes exhibited by horses restrained before the start of exercise, in which case it is generally regarded as a normal sign of impatience in an excitable animal (Cook 1979a). In both of these situations the headshaking behaviour should be considered a normal physiological response. However, a persistent tossing or shaking of the head, especially at exercise, is abnormal, and these horses are generally referred to as "headshakers".

EPIDEMIOLOGY

The precise incidence of headshaking in the equine population is unknown, but the disease is widely recognized throughout the country. Cook (1979a) noted a higher incidence among thoses trained for dressage, but in a more recent survey (Lane and Mair 1987) no such association could be shown, and the disease has been recognized in animals used for a variety of purposes including racing, showjumping, eventing, dressage, hunting, showing and long-distance riding. The problem is seen in all breeds and sexes.

The disease is frequently seasonal, both in onset and recurrence of signs:

(1) The peak periods of onset of headshaking are spring (March/April) and early summer (May/June), and the signs of disease generally regress spontaneously in the autumn and remain absent until the following spring.
(2) In a smaller proportion of cases the problem appears to be at its worst during the autumn, but again tends to disappear during the winter.
(3) In some horses signs may persist all year round, and in many of these the problem may have been noted to be seasonal for the first year or two, followed by the continuous presence of signs thereafter.

CLINICAL SIGNS

The signs of headshaking are observed at exercise, especially at the trot, but as the condition progresses they may be seen at other paces and at rest. The behaviour typically starts within five to 10 minutes of the start of exercise, i.e. when the horse has warmed up. The following signs are often observed.

(1) Intermittent, sudden and apparently involuntary head tossing or nodding movements of such an extravagant kind that both horse and rider can be thrown off balance.

(2)   The direction of the head movement is usually vertical although horizontal and rotary movements are sometimes observed.

(3)   In some cases an exaggerated upward motion of the head is accompanied by an extension and elevation of a forelimb.

(4)   Sneezing and snorting are frequently present, and many cases show evidence of nasal irritation, with attempts by the horse to rub its nose on a foreleg, the rider's leg, or on the ground.

(5)   Owners often describe their horses as behaving as if a bee is sitting on the end of the nose.

Once the signs of headshaking have begun during exercise they generally become progressively worse to the extent that, if the horse is kept working, the animal becomes very distressed and the behaviour seems almost maniacal. In these circumstances the horse is obviously a danger to both itself and its rider. On return to the stable many affected horses will continue to show signs of nasal irritation with snorting, twitching of the nostrils and rubbing of the nose.

The occurrence and severity of clinical signs often correlate with the weather conditions and the locality in which the horse is being exercised. Thus, the disease tends to be more pronounced on warm, sunny days, and is frequently at its worst when the horse is ridden near trees and hedgerows.

AETIOLOGY

There are many different underlying diseases which can result in the behavioural signs of headshaking. Since the problem is frequently unresponsive to therapy, there has been a tendency to regard headshaking as a stereotypic behaviour problem or a "vice". While this may be so in some cases, in the majority it is likely that the behaviour is secondary to an underlying disease mechanism that causes pain, irritation or discomfort.

A list of some of the possible causes of headshaking is shown in Table 6.1. The study by Lane and Mair (1987) concluded that the epidemiological and clinical features of the majority of cases are consistent with an allergic rhinitis,

Table 6.1 Problems that can be associated with headshaking in the horse.

Bit and tack problems

Respiratory tract
Allergic rhinitis
Vasomotor rhinitis
Paranasal sinus disease

Nervous system
Trigeminal neuralgia
Stereotypic behaviour abnormality
Vestibular syndrome

Ear
Psoroptic mange mites
Foreign bodies
Guttural pouch disease
Otitis interna

Eye (Fig. 6.2)
Photophobia
Iris cysts
Uveitis
Retinal lesions

Musculoskeletal system
Cervical vertebral pain
Myositis of the neck
Exostoses at occipital protuberance

Digestive system
Pain from bit impinging on diastema, tush or wolf teeth
Buccal ulceration
Periodontal disease
Dental periapical abscess

but this hypothesis has yet to be confirmed by specific immunological testing.

Anecdotal evidence from a number of sources suggests that the incidence of headshaking has been increasing during the past few years. A similar increase in the incidence of allergic diseases in man such as asthma and hay fever has been observed during this period. Strictly, hay fever refers to grass pollen allergy, whereas the term seasonal rhinitis covers reactions to other pollen types. Tree pollens often predominate in April and early May, before grass pollen levels peak in the first two weeks of June. Between July and September mould spores are more common. All of these pollens have been implicated in the aetiology of seasonal rhinitis in man, and a similar role in headshaking seems possible. Pollen from oil seed rape has recently been recognized as a cause of allergic disease in both man and the horse (Fig. 6.1). Rape has been cultivated increasingly in the UK since the late 1970s. The pollen does not seem to carry far on the wind and allergy may be a problem predominantly for people and animals living close to areas where rape is being cultivated.

INVESTIGATION

The investigation of the headshaker is often very time consuming, and frequently disappointing. It is only in a minority of cases that a precise diagnosis can be reached, and even if an abnormality is detected it is not always possible to establish its significance with respect to the headshaking. The costs of such investigations can be high and, in view of the distinct possibility that the results may be inconclusive, the procedure may be rendered economically unsatisfactory for the owner as well as scientifically unrewarding for the veterinary surgeon. A protocol for the suggested investigation is summarized in Table 6.2. The investigation should commence with a thorough appraisal of the history of the case, since this will often give clues as to the underlying aetiology.

(1) Cases of allergic rhinitis usually show signs that are seasonal, and affected animals are frequently sold during the winter months when the signs are absent.

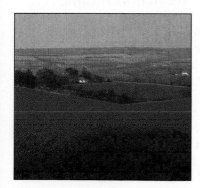

Fig. 6.1
Oil seed rape which has been grown in increasing quantities since the 1970s and has recently been recognized as an important potential allergen in man and the horse. There is much anecdotal evidence to link exposure to rape pollen with headshaking in certain horses.

Table 6.2 Investigation protocol for the headshaker.

Initial investigation	Further diagnostic procedures	
History		Diagnosis
Management tests (performed by owner)		Diagnosis
Clinical examination Respiratory tract	Endoscopy ⎱ Radiography ⎰	Diagnosis
Cranial nerves	Radiography (possibly under GA) ⎱ Infraorbital nerve block ⎰ CSF analysis	Diagnosis
Ears	Otoscopy (under GA) ⎱ Radiography (under GA) ⎰ Endoscopy (guttural pouches)	Diagnosis
Eyes	Ophthalmoscopy	Diagnosis
Musculoskeletal system	Radiography ⎱ Serum chemistry ⎰	Diagnosis
Digestive system	Radiograph (teeth)	Diagnosis

(2)   Most cases of allergic rhinitis begin during the spring, and some may follow on from a respiratory tract infection.
(3)   The importance of weather conditions and environment on the severity of clinical signs should be assessed; these factors are likely to have profound effects on cases of allergic rhinitis.
(4)   Horses with allergic rhinitis frequently demonstrate other immune-mediated problems such as chronic obstructive pulmonary disease, sweet itch and recurrent urticaria.

Intolerance of the bit or problems with the tack are frequently blamed as the cause of headshaking. With this in mind, the owner should be asked to perform various management tests to answer the following questions:

(1)   Do the signs of headshaking persist when the horse is exercised on the lunge, with or without a bit in its mouth, and with and without a saddle on its back?
(2)   Is the headshaking affected by riding the horse with different bits, or with a bitless bridle?

(3) Is the headshaking altered if the horse is ridden with a different saddle, or with no saddle?

Once bit and tack problems have been eliminated as the cause of headshaking, a thorough clinical examination of the patient should be performed, paying particular attention to examination of structures of the head and neck. Further diagnostic procedures such as endoscopic examination of the upper airways and guttural pouches, ophthalmoscopy, otoscopy and radiography may be indicated; some of these procedures may need to be performed under general anaesthesia.

Infraorbital nerve blocking (Fig. 6.3) is indicated in cases where trigeminal neuritis is suspected, or in order to try to assess the potential efficacy of infraorbital neurectomy for

(A)

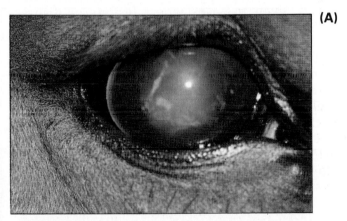

(B)

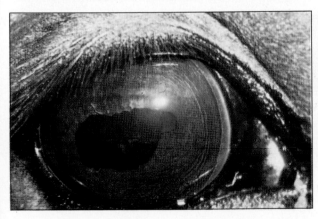

Fig. 6.2
Ocular conditions such as uveitis (A) and hyperplasia of the granulae iridica (B) are frequently blamed as potential causes of headshaking but, in practice, they are rarely identified in these cases.

treatment (see below). This nerve is a branch of the maxillary division of the trigeminal nerve, and is entirely sensory. Blocking the nerve will desensitize the upper lip and cheek, the nostrils and lower parts of the face. The nerve is easily blocked as it emerges from the infraorbital canal; it can be palpated if the band-like levator nasolabialis muscle is pushed dorsally. Approximately 5 ml of a local anaesthetic agent (such as 2 per cent lignocaine) should be injected around the nerve.

TREATMENT

The treatment of headshaking is complicated by the fact that, in most cases, a specific diagnosis of the underlying condition is never achieved. Even in cases where lesions or diseases are identified, it is not always possible to convincingly link them to the headshaker syndrome. For example, an animal affected by otitis externa due to the presence of *Psoroptes* species mites might be expected to shake its head in a horizontal manner with equal severity at rest and exercise; this is extremely unusual in the true headshaker, even in cases where such mites are identified. Likewise, it is difficult to explain the signs of apparent nasal irritation as a consequence of aural irritation. Ear mites have been reported to be present in up to 20 per cent of horses in Queensland, Australia, most of which show no clinical signs (Pascoe 1980). None the

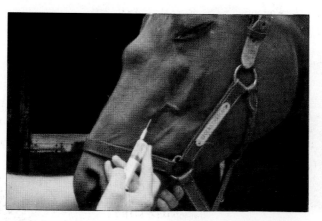

Fig. 6.3
Infraorbital nerve blocking will desensitize the upper lip and cheek, the nostril and lower parts of the face. The procedure is generally well accepted by the horse, and is indicated in cases where trigeminal neuritis is suspected or to assess the potential efficacy of infraorbital neurectomy.

less, the identification or suspicion of otitis externa and, or, ear mite infestation in a headshaking horse warrants appropriate treatment.

Cranial nerve dysfunction and cervical vertebral damage have been identified by a number of workers as causes of headshaking (Blythe and others 1984, Lane and Mair 1987), but such problems are rarely amenable to therapy. On the other hand, some ocular problems, such as melanotic iris cysts, and guttural pouch diseases, such as mycosis (Fig. 6.4), may be treatable, and cases of headshaking that have recovered after appropriate therapy for such diseases have been recorded (Lane and Mair 1987).

The seasonal nature of the headshaking problem in most cases of allergic rhinitis means that some owners may be willing to accept the fact that the horse is unrideable for part of the year. However, in practice this seems to be rarely acceptable. Another alternative is to completely alter the animal's environment and location in which it is ridden, but this is usually not possible. In some cases, alleviation of the signs (albeit temporarily) may be attained by riding the horse with a peice of muslin or fine mesh hanging from the bridle and falling over the nostrils.

Medical therapy of suspected allergic rhinitis cases has been largely unrewarding (Mair and others 1992). Treatment has been attempted in a number of cases by local therapy with inhaled sodium cromoglycate, or systemic therapy with corticosteroids or antihistamines, with very little success. A

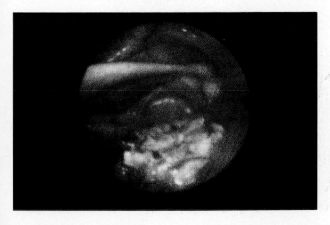

Fig. 6.4
Mycotic infection of the guttural pouches is another uncommon cause of headshaking.

better success rate has been achieved by using local (inhaled) beclomethasone, but the dosage and frequency of administration need to be modified to suit the individual case, and the treatment may become unacceptably expensive. Surgical treatment by infraorbital neurectomy (Fig. 6.5) has been suggested for many years, but there is little published information concerning its efficacy. In our experience here at Bristol, this somewhat speculative procedure is probably effective in no more than 30 per cent to 40 per cent of cases, but where a favourable response is achieved it is often complete. The nerves are sectioned as they leave the infraorbital canals, and the procedure is best performed under general anaesthesia to ensure complete sectioning of the wide, band-like nerve bundles. The ends of the nerves should be treated by cryotherapy to limit the risk of re-innervation or neuroma formation.

Rubbing of the nostrils and side of face is a not infrequent complication of this surgery, but in most cases this is a

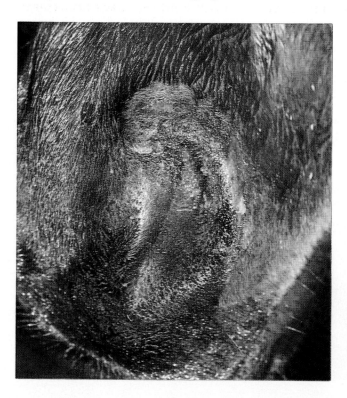

Fig. 6.5
Nasal pruritus is frequent temporary complication of infraorbital neurectomy.

temporary problem; some horses may take a period of a few days to a few weeks to fully adjust to the loss of sensation around the upper lip and cheek.

Alternative forms of therapy may be worth considering in some cases. Acupuncture has apparently been successful in a limited number of horses.

INSURANCE CONSIDERATIONS

Headshakers are often the subjects of loss of use insurance claims. Whenever the attending veterinary surgeon is satisfied that the horse is dangerous or unreasonably difficult to ride, a claim may be justly supported. Some insurance companies may request treatment by infraorbital neurectomy before any such claim is considered. Since most headshakers are asymptomatic at rest in the stable or when grazing, claims for destruction on humanitarian grounds are usually inappropriate.

REFERENCES AND FURTHER READING

Blythe, L. L., Watrous, B. J., Schmitz, J. A. & Kaneps, A. J. (1984). *Journal of the American Veterinary Medical Association* **185**, 775.
Cook, W. R. (1979a). *Equine Practice* **1**, 9.
Cook, W. R. (1979b). *Equine Practice* **1**, 36.
Cook, W. R. (1979d). *Equine Practice* **2**, 31.
Lane, J. G. & Mair, T. S. (1987). *Equine Veterinary Journal* **19**, 331.
Mair, T. S., Howarth, S. & Lane, J. G. (1992). *Equine Veterinary Journal* suppl. **11**, 10–12.
Pascoe, R. R. (1980). *Veterinary Record* **107**, 234.

CHAPTER 7

Differential Diagnosis of Hepatic Disorders in Horses

ELSPETH M. MILNE

INTRODUCTION

The remarkable capacity of the liver to regenerate ensures that mild damage is rarely associated with clinical signs and hepatic disease may not be suspected until signs of liver failure develop. At this stage, the prognosis tends to be poor, regardless of the initiating cause.

Hepatic disease may be divided into primary conditions which mainly affect the liver and secondary conditions where the liver is affected as part of a more generalized disorder (Table 7.1).

GENERAL CLINICAL SIGNS

The liver has a major role in carbohydrate, protein and lipid metabolism. Soluble carbohydrates from the small intestine may be stored as hepatic glycogen while glucose is also produced by gluconeogenesis using glycogen, amino acids and certain fatty acids as precursors. Many important proteins are synthesized in the liver, for example some clotting factors and albumin. Bile production and storage of the fat-soluble

Table 7.1 Primary and secondary causes of hepatic disorders.

Primary	Secondary
Toxic	*Metabolic* (fatty liver)
Ragwort poisoning	Equine hyperlipaemia
Mycotoxins, e.g. aflatoxin	Hyperadrenocorticism
Acute hepatitis (Theiler's disease)	Anorexia/starvation
Neoplastic	*Neoplastic*
Hepatic carcinoma	Metastases, e.g. lymphosarcoma,
Bile duct carcinoma	squamous cell carcinoma,
	adenocarcinoma
Bacterial	*Bacterial*
Leptospirosis	Liver abscesses
Cholangiohepatitis	
Parasitic	*Parasitic*
Liver fluke (*Fasciola hepatica*)	Obstruction of bile ducts by
Echinococcus granulosus	*Parascaris equorum*
Others	
Obstructive cholelithiasis	
Congenital portosystemic vascular	
shunts	

vitamins A, D and E are essential hepatic functions together with metabolism of toxic products such as urea. In view of its many functions, hepatic failure produces a variety of clinical signs.

Liver failure may become apparent when at least half of the hepatocytes are damaged or destroyed. Prior to this stage, reduction in feed intake and weight loss may both occur, but they are often not severe enough for the owner to seek veterinary help. Jaundice is a variable feature, most consistently seen in acute hepatitis and in conditions where cholestasis is severe. It should be borne in mind, however, that anorexia for any reason is the most common cause of jaundiced mucous membranes in the horse. Once hepatic function is compromised, weight loss occurs and hepatic encephalopathy may develop in association with the neurotoxic effects of hyperammonaemia and a decreased ratio of branched chain to aromatic amino acids in the serum. This is manifest by behavioural and neurological changes including dullness, a vacant expression, yawning, ataxia, tremors and, in severe cases, circling, head-pressing (Fig. 7.1) and occasionally aggression.

Photosensitive dermatitis may affect non-pigmented or thinly haired areas of skin exposed to sunlight, usually the muzzle and lower limbs. Initially the areas appear erythematous, then progress to hair loss, crusting and irritation. Photosensitization is caused by failure of the liver to metabolize phylloerythrin, a breakdown product of chlorophyll metabolism.

Abdominal pain, manifest as mild to severe colic, is often present. This is generally considered to be associated with hepatomegaly, but secondary gastric impaction has recently been recognized in hepatic failure caused by ragwort poisoning. Polydipsia and polyuria are inconsistent findings. The faeces may be of a cowpat consistency, either intermittently or continuously, or may be normal.

Impaired blood coagulation caused by failure of the liver to produce clotting factors may result in petechial haemorrhages in the oral and vulval mucosae, are especially common and in the equine hyperlipaemia syndrome. Severe haemorrhage is rare. Ascites is also uncommon and subcutaneous oedema inconsistent. Where the latter occurs it is usually seen in the lower limbs, brisket and ventral abdomen.

In the case of secondary hepatic failure, other signs associated with the systemic disease are likely to be seen. Foals with liver abscesses associated with *Rhodococcus equi* infection, for example, may exhibit respiratory signs while cases with metastatic neoplasia may show signs associated with the primary lesion.

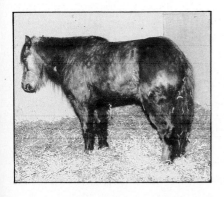

Fig. 7.1
A pony exhibiting severe depression and head-pressing behaviour associated with hepatic encephalopathy.

DIAGNOSTIC AIDS

Hepatic disease is difficult to diagnose by clinical signs alone and the use of laboratory tests is therefore of paramount importance. However, the results of such tests depend on the nature, duration and severity of the damage and tests measuring cell damage may give results at variance with those tests used to measure liver function.

TESTS FOR LIVER DAMAGE (Table 7.2)

Liver-derived serum enzyme concentrations are valuable indicators of hepatic damage and may be raised prior to the onset of signs of hepatic failure. Sorbitol dehydrogenase (SDH) and glutamate dehydrogenase (GLDH) are relatively liver-specific intracellular enzymes which are released from damaged hepatocytes, peak levels occurring one to two days

Table 7.2 Normal values*.

Test of liver damage	
Glutamate dehydrogenase	1–12 iu/litre
Gamma-glutamyl transpeptidase	13–44 iu/litre
Alkaline phosphatase	84–180 iu/litre
Aspartate aminotransferase	258–554 iu/litre
Total bilirubin	17–34 μmol/litre
Tests of liver damage and function	
Bile acids	0.8–15.4 μmol/litre
Ammonia	15–90 μmol/litre
Test of liver function	
BSP dye clearance ($T\frac{1}{2}$)	2.0–3.7 minutes
Non-specific tests	
Glucose	2.8–5.5 mmol/litre
Total protein	58–75 g/litre
Albumin	23–35 g/litre
Globulin	30–58 g/litre
Prothrombin time	9–12 seconds
Cholesterol	2.3–3.6 mmol/litre
Triglyceride	0.2–0.9 mmol/litre
Urea	2.5–8.3 mmol/litre

* R(D)SVS Clinical Laboratory (D. L. Doxey, unpublished).

after a single insult. Their short serum half-life (12 to 14 hours) means that if they are consistently elevated, active damage is continuing. SDH has the disadvantage of being unstable in blood samples. Lactate dehydrogenase (LDH) and aspartate aminotransferase (AST) are also increased in the serum during hepatocellular damage and have a longer serum half-life. They have the disadvantage that they are not liver-specific but are useful in following progress when liver damage has been detected by some other means. The specificity of LDH can be improved by quantitation of its isoenzymes in serum. Serum alkaline phosphatase (AP) and gamma-glutamyl transpeptidase (GGT) are mainly found in the biliary tree and are elevated when bile flow is impaired due to intrahepatic or post-hepatic lesions. AP is not a liver-specific enzyme and is not a reliable indicator of liver damage in horses when used on its own even when its liver isoenzyme is assayed. Infiltrative lesions do not induce the large increases in AP seen in dogs with similar problems. GGT is more specific and sensitive especially in very severe acute damage or in chronic liver damage where active hepatocellular disruption is minimal and SDH or GLDH may not be markedly elevated. It is advisable to assay at least two liver enzymes in view of the different circumstances associated with their increase in the serum, e.g. GLDH and GGT. Serial determinations help to assess progression of the disease.

Serum bilirubin is a useful indicator of cholestasis and the largest increases are likely to occur when there is marked cholestasis; for example, in lesions which obstruct the bile ducts, levels of 400 μmol/litre may be reached. Horses are unusual in that most of the serum bilirubin is unconjugated in pre-, intra- and post-hepatic jaundice and determination of the proportion of conjugated and unconjugated serum bilirubin is of little value in indicating the type of jaundice present. Furthermore, anorexia for a few days can increase serum bilirubin to as high as 80 to 90 μmol/litre in the absence of hepatic disease.

TESTS FOR LIVER DAMAGE AND FUNCTION
(Table 7.2)

Some tests can be used to assess both damage and function in the sense that a single test result indicates whether, as a result of cell damage, the liver is able to perform normal functions such as the removal of bile acids from the circulation. Serum bile acids appear to be valuable indicators of cholestatic disease in hepatic failure in the horse and the test is now widely offered by laboratories.

Blood ammonia levels may be raised due to failure of the liver to convert ammonia to urea, but it is not invariably so. Increased levels therefore provide supportive evidence for hepatic damage and failure but normal levels do not preclude this. Ammonia tends to be elevated in acute, severe liver failure or in the late stages of chronic liver failure. A concurrent decrease in blood urea may sometimes be detected.

NON-SPECIFIC TESTS (Table 7.2)

Blood glucose is usually normal in hepatic failure but a few horses will develop signs of hypoglycaemia. The latter is particularly common in the equine hyperlipaemia syndrome although hepatic failure is not the major cause of the hypoglycaemia in this condition.

The clotting factors II (prothrombin), V, VII, IX and X may be reduced. Clearly, information regarding impaired coagulation is important if liver biopsy is to be carried out and prothrombin time is the most readily available test for this purpose.

Serum protein changes are not specific but may provide supportive evidence of hepatic damage and impaired function. Serum albumin may be reduced in the later stages of hepatic disease due to impaired synthesis but there is often a concurrent increase in beta globulins so that total serum proteins may not necessarily be reduced. Serum albumin is also markedly reduced in a variety of non-hepatic disorders. Below a critical albumin level of approximately 15 g/litre, subcutaneous oedema or ascites may be observed. Gamma-globulins may also be increased in inflammatory conditions such as liver abscesses or cholangiohepatitis.

Routine haematology is generally unhelpful for the specific detection of hepatic disease although it has some value in determining the cause. Horses with liver abscesses or cholangiohepatitis may have a neutrophilia with or without a monocytosis. Some cases of hepatic failure show mild anaemia and occasionally severe intravascular haemolysis occurs resulting in profound haemolytic anaemia.

Urine analysis may be a useful preliminary screening test. Bilirubinuria may be detected if there is a significant hyperbilirubinaemia, despite the fact that most of the serum bilirubin is unconjugated and therefore albumin-bound. Bilirubin gives the urine a brown colour. On the rare occasions where intravascular haemolysis occurs in association with hepatic failure, marked haemoglobinuria with free haemo-globin and haemoglobin casts may be present and the urine will be discoloured red.

Peritoneal fluid examination is not particularly helpful in confirming the presence of hepatic failure but should be carried out as many of the differential diagnoses of hepatic failure, e.g. other causes of chronic abdominal pain or weight loss, result in changes in peritoneal fluid. In general, peritoneal fluid is dark yellow or orange in hepatic failure due to an increase in bilirubin but, if ascites has developed, fluid with the characteristics of a transudate will be obtained. An increase in protein and total white blood cell count may be seen in liver abscessation if peritonitis has resulted and, occasionally, neoplastic cells can be detected in primary or secondary hepatic neoplasia.

TESTS FOR LIVER FUNCTION (Table 7.2)

An exogenous substance, such as a dye, is administered to the patient and the ability of the liver to eliminate the substance may be assessed quantitatively. These tests require two or more blood samples at timed intervals and the best known in the UK is the bromosulphthalein clearance test.

Bromosulphthalein (BSP) clearance is a valuable test for assessing liver function in horses. BSP injected intravenously is taken up by the liver, conjugated with glutathione and excreted in the bile. It has been stated that bile acid assay is a replacement for BSP clearance but this is not the case as the two assays test different metabolic functions.

Procedure for BSP clearance test

(1)   Prepare 1 g BSP in 20 ml distilled water and sterilize by autoclave (some laboratories will provide sterile BSP).
(2)   Inject the solution as a bolus into one jugular vein, starting a stop-watch when midway through the injection.
(3)   At 3 minutes collect a 7 ml heparinized blood sample from the *other* jugular vein.
(4)   At 6 minutes collect a second heparinized blood sample from the same vein as the previous sample.

If the blood samples are to be posted to the laboratory, the plasma should be harvested first. The timing of samples need not be exactly 3 and 6 minutes but the exact time of collection must be noted. The laboratory will calculate the BSP clearance as a half-clearance time. The normal half-clearance time is 2.0 to 3.7 minutes. If the value exceeds 4 minutes, suspicion of hepatic failure is present and times exceeding 5 minutes are highly significant. Hyperbilirubinaemia associated with anorexia and any cause of a decrease in hepatic blood flow may increase the half-clearance time but rarely to more than 5 minutes.

LIVER BIOPSY

Most of the tests described above are only of value in detecting the presence of liver disease while liver biopsy clearly can provide a definitive diagnosis in some cases. Most equine liver disorders are diffuse, e.g. diffuse neoplasia, ragwort poisoning and fatty degeneration so that liver biopsy can be particularly useful in this species. Focal lesions are easily missed.

Before carrying out liver biopsy, prothrombin time, whole blood clotting time and thrombocyte count should be measured. The former is particularly important and if prothrombin time exceeds 20 seconds, one to two litres of platelet-rich equine plasma should be transfused just before attempting biopsy. Although rare, major haemorrhage is a potential complication of liver biopsy. Other complications such as introduction of infection and penetration of organs other than the liver can be the result of poor technique.

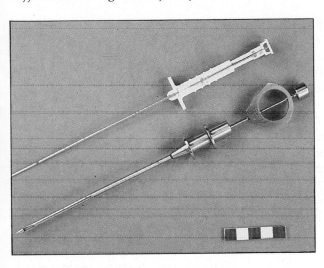

Fig. 7.2
Liver biopsy needles.
(Top) 14 cm resterilizable
liver biopsy needle
(Economy instruments).
(Bottom) 15.2 cm-cannula
Tru-Cut disposable biopsy
needle (Travenol
Laboratories).

Procedure for liver biopsy

An imaginary line is drawn from the point of the shoulder
to the tuber coxae and the site identified where this line
crosses the 14th intercostal space on the right side. The
site is surgically prepared and local anaesthetic injected
subcutaneously and down to the parietal pleura in the 14th
intercostal space. A stab incision is made through the skin
close to the anterior edge of the 15th rib with a No 15 scalpel
blade and the biopsy needle (Figs 7.2 and 7.3) slowly inserted

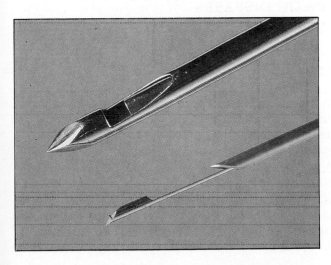

Fig. 7.3
Specimen collection slots
on the biopsy needles
shown in Fig. 7.2.

at right angles to the skin. It will pass through the diaphragm when the needle will move with respiration. As it is advanced further the resistance of the liver capsule can be felt. The needle is advanced a few centimetres into the parenchyma and the sample collected. The sample should be carefully removed from the needle and placed in 10 per cent formol saline. The skin wound can be sutured or covered with a dressing and the horse kept quiet and watched for signs of haemorrhage for the next few hours. Tetanus antitoxin should be given if necessary.

OTHER DIAGNOSTIC AIDS

Transabdominal ultrasound is now proving valuable for assessing the size, shape, position and texture of the liver. Choleliths are highly reflective on ultrasonic examination and primary and secondary neoplasia and fibrosis in chronic liver disease have been detected. Ultrasound is also extremely valuable for guided liver biopsy, especially in facilitating biopsy of focal lesions.

SPECIFIC HEPATIC CONDITIONS IN THE HORSE

PRIMARY HEPATIC DISEASES

Ragwort poisoning

Poisoning with plants containing pyrrolizidine alkaloids is the major cause of liver disease in horses in the UK and is caused by ingestion of ragwort (*Senecio jacobaea*) at pasture or in contaminated hay. There is usually a history of long term exposure to the plant. The clinical signs are slow to develop and acute poisoning is rare but even in chronic cases signs of hepatic failure may appear suddenly. There may be a history of gradual weight loss, a decrease in appetite and sometimes recurrent bouts of photosensitization (Fig. 7.4) before terminal hepatic failure develops when signs including

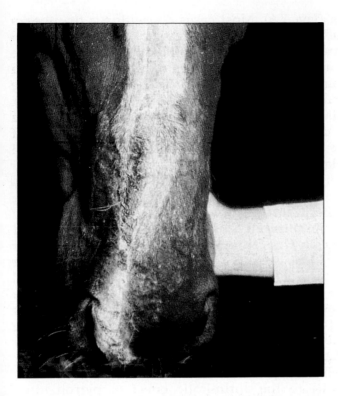

Fig. 7.4
Photosensitive
dermatitis affecting
the non-pigmented
and thinly haired
areas.

weight loss, hepatic encephalopathy, variable jaundice (Fig. 7.5), photosensitization, constipation, diarrhoea or abdominal pain will be seen. Secondary gastric impaction may be a terminal complication and gastric rupture is sometimes the

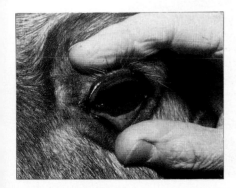

Fig. 7.5
Jaundice of the conjunctiva.

cause of death (Fig. 7.6). Most cases die within a few weeks of the onset of signs of hepatic failure.

Of the laboratory tests, serum GGT is the most sensitive indicator of the liver damage and will be raised prior to and during the stage of hepatic failure with levels often reaching 1000 iu/litre. AP is also likely to be markedly increased and may reach 3000 iu/litre. Levels of enzymes indicative of hepatocellular damage (e.g. GLDH and SDH) are variable and depend on the number of hepatocytes which remain and are therefore available to be damaged. Bile acids are consistently raised but total protein, albumin and globulin concentrations are variable. Blood ammonia levels are increased in some cases but can be normal even when hepatic encephalopathy is present. Serum bilirubin levels are also variable but a mild to moderate increase is common. BSP clearance is invariably impaired with a half-clearance time of 15 minutes or more at the terminal stage.

Liver biopsy is the only means of making a definitive ante mortem diagnosis as the clinical signs and laboratory findings are similar to other types of chronic hepatic failure. There will be evidence of degeneration and necrosis of hepatocytes and their replacement with fibrous tissue (Fig. 7.7), bile duct proliferation and the presence of characteristic megalocytes which occur due to the antimitotic effect of pyrrolizidine alkaloids on the hepatocytes. At post mortem examination, the liver is of a normal or reduced size (Fig. 7.8) with a

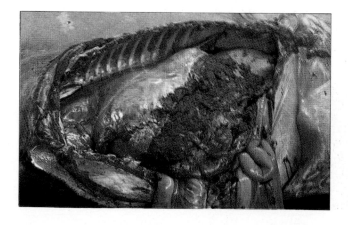

Fig. 7.6
Gastric dilation and rupture may occur secondary to ragwort poisoning.

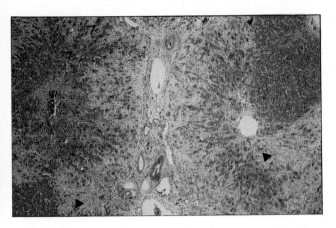

Fig. 7.7
Photomicrograph of a
section of liver from a
case of ragwort
poisoning showing
loss of hepatocytes
and replacement with
fibrous tissue which
is stained green
(solid arrows) and
megalocytosis (open
arrows). Masson's
trichrome × 20.

nodular surface, a firm consistency and a colour varying from yellow to greenish-brown or brown.

Once hepatic failure develops, the prognosis is hopeless.

Aflatoxicosis

Ingestion of mouldy feeds contaminated with *Aspergillus* species of fungi can cause clinical signs and laboratory findings similar to those of ragwort poisoning. Histopathology is also similar to that of ragwort poisoning although megalocytosis is generally much less marked than in ragwort

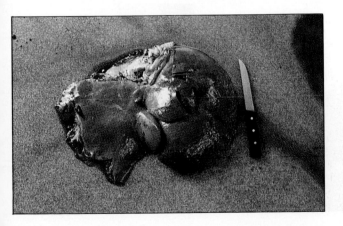

Fig. 7.8
Affected liver
demonstrating
reduction in size, a
nodular surface and
a pale brown
coloration in ragwort
poisoning.

poisoning and the latter is, in any case, a much more common condition.

Primary hepatic neoplasia

Primary neoplasia is rare with hepatocellular carcinomas being most commonly encountered. They are single or may metastasize within the liver and into the peritoneal cavity and lungs. Clinical signs of hepatic failure may develop if the lesions are extensive or obstruct the bile ducts. The laboratory findings vary with the size, site and number of lesions and the most marked changes, similar to those found in obstructive cholelithiasis will occur if bile duct obstruction occurs. Occasionally, neoplastic cells can be detected in peritoneal fluid. Liver biopsy may be valuable but focal lesions can be missed. Transabdominal ultrasound seems particularly useful in detecting lesions and can also be used for guided biopsy.

Leptospirosis

Serological evidence of leptospiral infection has been described in 35 per cent of 500 clinically normal horses in England in one survey (Hathaway and others 1981) but clinical signs of the disease are rare. These include pyrexia, jaundice, petechiation of the mucous membranes (Fig. 7.9), haematuria and sometimes bilateral conjunctivitis, CNS signs and acute renal failure.

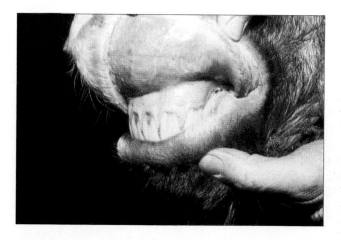

Fig. 7.9
Petechial
haemorrhages of the
oral mucous
membranes.

Full laboratory investigations do not seem to have been undertaken in the cases described, but markedly raised liver enzymes would be expected in the serum, particularly SDH and GLDH, indicative of acute hepatocellular damage, together with high serum bilirubin levels.

Paired serum samples, two to three weeks apart, will show a rising titre, most commonly to antigens from the *icterohaemorrhagiae* and *australis* subgroups.

Cholangiohepatitis

Cholangiohepatitis is very rare in horses in the UK. The disease seems to be caused by reflux of intestinal contents containing bacteria into the biliary system concurrent with biliary obstruction. Chronic weight loss and colic just before death have been described and laboratory findings include an increase in serum AP and GGT and a marked hyperbilirubinaemia together with an increase in urine bilirubin.

Gross hepatomegaly occurs in acute cases and the liver is pale and soft with multiple septic foci. In chronic cases nodular regeneration may be seen.

Liver fluke

Fasciola hepatica infection is a rare cause of serious hepatic disease in horses. Equines grazing wet pastures during the summer are at risk especially where there is contamination by affected sheep and cattle, and hepatic failure associated with scar tissue formation and nodular areas of regeneration may occur. The fluke larvae cause hepatocellular damage as they migrate through the liver parenchyma and the adults cause fibrosis and partial obstruction of the bile ducts. During migration, SDH and GLDH may be preferentially increased while AP and GGT may be highest in patent infections. Patent infections can also be detected by identification of fluke eggs in the faeces.

Echinococcus granulosus

Ten per cent of British horses are said to harbour cysts of the tapeworm *Echinococcus granulosus* which are distinct from the sheep strain. Foxhounds are the main definitive host of the equine strain. Multiple cysts may be seen in the liver (Fig. 7.10), and occasionally lungs, ranging from a few millimetres to several centimetres in diameter. They are usually incidental findings but can cause hepatic failure if present in large numbers. Cysts may be detected by ultrasound followed by guided aspiration.

Obstructive cholelithiasis

Biliary calculi are rare in the horse. They may be single or multiple and are often associated with recurrent colic, weight loss and jaundice. Laboratory findings suggest cholestasis. Histopathology of the liver biopsies may be non-specific with portal fibrosis, bile duct proliferation, cholestasis and groups of necrotic hepatocytes at the periphery of lobules. It is difficult to distinguish between cholelithiasis and other forms of biliary obstruction, but biliary calculi have been detected ante mortem by transabdominal ultrasound.

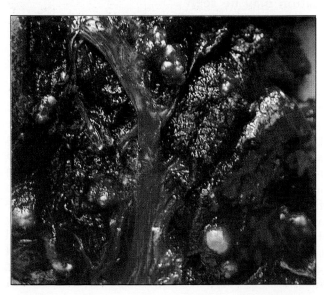

Fig. 7.10
Cut surface of equine liver with multiple cysts of *Echinococcus granulosus.*

Portosystemic vascular shunts

Congenital abnormalities of the portal vein are much rarer in horses than in small animals and only a few cases have been reported. The foals may present with signs of depression and hepatic encephalopathy at up to a few months old. Laboratory investigation is likely to reveal normal or mildly raised GGT and AP but increased serum bilirubin, bile acids and ammonia, decreased blood urea and a prolonged BSP half-clearance time (seven to nine minutes). Liver biopsy will reveal widespread hepatocyte atrophy and many small arterioles in the portal triads. The history, clinical signs and laboratory and biopsy findings are strongly suggestive of the condition.

Acute hepatitis (Theiler's disease)

Theiler's disease is an acute hepatitis of uncertain aetiology in adult horses and appears to be a problem mainly in North America. Cases have occurred after the administration of equine serum products but a viral aetiology has also been suggested. The clinical signs are typical of acute hepatic failure and include signs of hepatic encephalopathy, abdominal pain, photosensitization and severe jaundice. Marked increases in serum SDH and GLDH are expected although GGT and AP may also be elevated. Serum bilirubin is generally higher than in chronic hepatic failure and bilirubinuria will occur. Bile acids are likely to be elevated, as in chronic hepatic failure.

The history, clinical signs and laboratory findings are often strongly suggestive of this condition but definitive ante mortem diagnosis can only be made by liver biopsy which will reveal degeneration and necrosis of hepatocytes, especially in the centrilobular and mid-zonal areas.

SECONDARY HEPATIC DISEASES

Anorexia

Mild jaundice is a very common finding in many anorexic horses, especially those with gastrointestinal disorders which reduce motility. It is not a cause of hepatic failure unless other predisposing factors precipitate the hyperlipaemia syndrome. Such animals will show mild hyperbilirubinaemia and normal or slightly increased liver enzyme levels. Serum proteins, blood ammonia, clotting factors and BSP clearance are unaffected. Serum triglycerides and cholesterol show mild increases but both parameters are usually less than 5 mmol/litre.

Equine hyperlipaemia syndrome

Equine hyperlipaemia is a metabolic disorder with a high mortality associated with development of a negative energy balance because of a decrease in food intake. Ninety per cent of cases are seen in mares in late pregnancy or early lactation. Transportation, parasitism, starvation or intercurrent disease can be initiating factors. Small, fat, pony breeds, especially Shetlands, are predisposed. There is usually a recent history of one of the initiating factors mentioned above and clinical signs may include dullness progressing to severe depression, inappetence, weight loss, muscular tremors and weak, ataxic gait. Ventral oedema, jaundice, petechial haemorrhages, diarrhoea and behavioural changes suggestive of hepatic encephalopathy may also be seen. Affected animals tend to chew slowly and some appear to be dysphagic. Abdominal pain may occur, probably due to hepatomegaly. Death usually occurs within 10 days of the onset of signs.

The aetiology is multifactorial and is considered to involve an increased demand for glucose together with a decreased intake, resulting in rapid fat mobilization. Insulin resistance in obese or pregnant ponies exacerbates the problem by decreasing uptake of mobilized fat from the circulation.

Laboratory investigation is very valuable in diagnosing this condition. Liver enzymes indicative of acute hepatocellular damage (SDH, GLDH) and cholestasis (AP, GGT) are usually markedly increased together with moderate increases in serum bilirubin and bile acids. Prothrombin time is sometimes prolonged. Serum samples have a milky or fluorescent appearance due to their high lipid content. Serum triglyceride levels are in the order of five to 50 mmol/litre and cholesterol levels reach five to 13 mmol/litre which are much higher than those seen in anorexia or simple starvation of a few days' duration. Hypoglycaemia and hypoalbuminaemia are common and BSP clearance is usually prolonged.

Liver biopsy may show severe fatty change and at post mortem examination hepatomegaly is found and fatty change in all parenchymatous organs is usually present. Hepatic rupture has been described as a cause of death in some cases. Vascular thrombosis may occur in the lung, kidneys and brain.

The history, clinical signs and laboratory findings are diagnostic when considered together.

Liver abscesses

Liver abscesses may occur following umbilical infections in foals, as part of a specific systemic disease such as *Rhodococcus equi* or *Actinobacillus equuli* infections in older foals or following strangles (*Streptococcus equi*) in young adults. There is likely to be a history of initial acute infection and clinical signs related to the systemic disease. Animals with liver, or other chronic abscesses, are likely to show weight loss and sometimes recurrent pyrexia and abdominal pain. Liver abscesses are rarely a cause of hepatic failure unless they are widespread or obstruct the major bile ducts. Depending on their number and site, however, they may cause an increase in liver enzymes or, if obstructing the bile ducts, a marked increase in serum bilirubin, bile acids, AP and GGT and the presence of increased urine bilirubin. Laboratory tests which detect inflammation or response to infection help to differentiate the condition from other forms of chronic liver disease, e.g. there may be a neutrophilia with a variable monocytosis and serum globulins and acute phase proteins such as fibrinogen may be increased. Blood culture and peritoneal fluid examination may also be of value. Lesions may be identified by ultrasound but "blind" liver biopsy is hazardous because of the risk of rupturing an abscess resulting in peritonitis.

Multi miliary liver abscesses occur in Tyzzer's disease (*Bacillus piliformis* infection) in foals of a few weeks of age but such animals are often found dead or die after a short illness with pyrexia, jaundice, recumbency, dyspnoea and convulsions. At post mortem examination, necrotizing enteritis and multifocal hepatic necrosis with polymorph infiltration may be identified. The bacilli may be demonstrated in the cytoplasm of hepatocytes using specific staining techniques.

Secondary neoplasia

A variety of neoplastic lesions may metastasize to the liver, e.g. lymphosarcoma, squamous cell carcinoma and adenocarcinoma. The first is the most common tumour. Unless they are very extensive or obstruct the bile ducts, the horse is unlikely to be presented with signs referable to hepatic involvement. Laboratory findings similar to those of cholelithiasis may be seen if bile duct obstruction occurs.

Hyperadrenocorticism (Fig. 7.11)

Hyperadrenocorticism secondary to pituitary neoplasia is an uncommon but well documented condition of older horses. The main clinical findings are chronic weight loss, growth of a long curly hair coat (hirsutism), alopecia and a "pot-bellied" appearance. As in dogs, glucocorticoid hepatopathy may occur with a mild to marked increase in serum AP and GGT. Mild hyperbilirubinaemia may be present and hyperglycaemia is

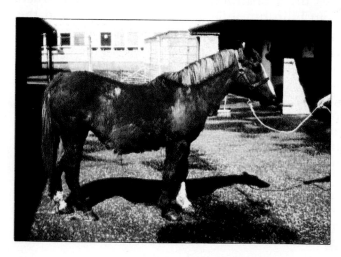

Fig. 7.11
Hyperadrenocorticism.

common. Liver biopsy will only reveal fatty infiltration and diagnosis depends on the use of dexamethasone suppression and ACTH stimulation tests.

CONCLUSIONS

There are a large number of conditions which cause hepatic dysfunction or failure in the horse. It is not difficult to detect liver damage but obtaining a definitive diagnosis can be difficult and meticulous clinical examination together with logical laboratory investigation is required. The importance of liver biopsy cannot be overemphasized and it is the only means of making an ante mortem diagnosis in many conditions. Transabdominal ultrasound has great potential as a diagnostic aid in hepatic disease.

ACKNOWLEDGEMENTS

Mr D. Collie, Dr D. L. Doxey, Miss A. McDonnell and Mr J. S. D. Ritchie kindly supplied some of the photographs.

FURTHER READING

Carlson, G. P. (1982). *Equine Medicine and Surgery*, 3rd edn, Vol. 1. Santa Barbara, California, American Veterinary Publications, p. 633.
Hathaway, S. C., Little, T. W. A., Finch, S. M. & Stevens, A. E. (1981). *Veterinary Record* **108**, 396.
Robinson, N. E. (1987). *Current Therapy in Equine Medicine*, 2nd edn. Philadelphia, W. B. Saunders.

CHAPTER 8

Equine Pituitary Neoplasia

ROBERT EUSTACE

INTRODUCTION

Despite demonstrating obvious abnormalities of clinical appearance, both the dog and the pony (Fig. 8.1) are suffering from the same condition: Cushing's syndrome (hyperadrenalcorticism). *Hyperadrenalcorticism produces the opposite changes in hair coat in the two species.* In equines this condition is always secondary to an adenoma of the pars intermedia of the pituitary gland (Figs 8.2 and 8.3), whereas in the dog the syndrome may be primarily of adrenal origin. Failure to shed the hair coat or the development of a matted or abnormally long coat for the breed of animal in an aged equine are strongly suggestive of a pituitary tumour.

Such cases always develop laminitis if they live long enough. They may become immunosuppressed and subject to a variety of parasitic or infectious agents such as helminthiasis or pneumonia. Many cases show muscle loss and become polydipsic and polyphagic; they may be diabetic. A curious peri-orbital swelling is commonly seen giving the eyes a protuberant appearance.

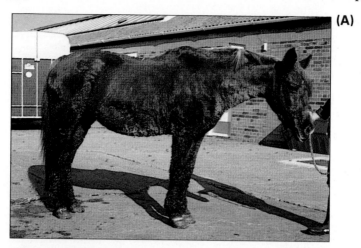

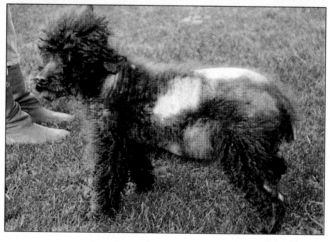

Fig. 8.1
Cushing's syndrome produces opposite changes in hair coat in the horse (A) and dog (B) (photo, Tim Gruffydd-Jones).

CONFIRMATORY TESTS

A plethora of tests have been used singly and in combination to try to confirm the diagnosis of pituitary neoplasia.

(1)   Single samples for resting cortisol or insulin concentrations are of no diagnostic value due to diurnal rhythm and normal wide variation between animals.
(2)   Cortisol assay using the ACTH stimulation test can be used for confirmation; however, there is a risk of inducing

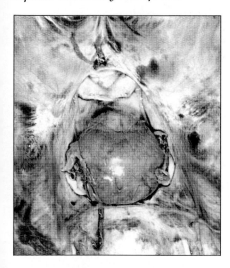

Fig. 8.2
Neoplastic equine pituitary gland left in the cranium following rupture of the infundibulum during removal of the brain.

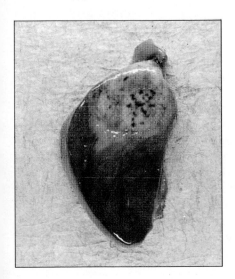

Fig. 8.3
Cut surface of the pituitary gland after sagittal sectioning to show the neoplasm.

or worsening a laminitic condition. Normal animals show an 80 per cent increase in cortisol concentration 2 hours after injecting 1 mg (100 iu) ACTH (Synacthen) intravenously (Eiler and others 1979). Pituitary tumour cases show a much greater response due to adrenal cortex hyperplasia.

(3)   Dexamethasone suppression test. Again this has the risk of inducing laminitis in the animal and is not recommended by this author. Normal animals show a 50 per cent decrease

in serum cortisol two hours following an intramuscular injection of 10 mg dexamethasone, the concentrations not returning to normal for at least 24 hours. Pituitary tumour cases may show no decrease in serum cortisol, or a much reduced decrease, and a return to baseline before 24 hours has elapsed following dexamethasone injection.

(4) The combined dexamethasone suppression and ACTH stimulation test, although more simple and quicker, is not recommended as the response to dexamethasone is not evaluated adequately.

(5) Intravenous glucose tolerance testing can be used (0.5 g glucose/kg body weight). Normal animals' glucose concentrations return to pre-test values within 60 minutes whereas pituitary tumour animals' glucose concentrations may remain elevated for up to 3 hours (Garcia and Beech 1986). Concurrent measurement of serum insulin concentrations during the above test may show pre-test hyperinsulinaemia and a much reduced insulin response to the glucose injection in pituitary tumour cases.

(6) A *safer alternative*, and the one test that this author recommends, is to assay for cortisol before intravenous injection of 1 mg thyroid releasing hormone (TRH;Roche) and at 15 and 60 minutes thereafter. Pituitary adenoma cases show an increase in cortisol of aproximately 90 per cent above baseline, at 15 minutes, compared to a rise of approximately 17 per cent in the normal animal (Beech and Garcia 1985). The cortisol concentration returns to baseline values at 60 minutes in the normal animal but may remain elevated at around 55 per cent above baseline in pituitary tumour cases.

The reliability of this test in donkeys is currently under evaluation; from preliminary results the cortisol response following the standard 1 mg dose of TRH appears higher in this species.

TREATMENT

Some temporary improvement in the clinical condition of such cases has resulted following treatment with cyproheptadine (Periactin;MSD). However, at best this results in a temporary improvement in the clinical condition of the animal, and it has no curative effect on the tumour. Many cases show no improvement following this treatment.

SUMMARY

In some animals this benign neoplasm seems to result in little disability other than the change in the haircoat. In other more advanced cases recurrent episodes of laminitis result or the animal may eventually succumb to an overwhelming systemic infection. However, many cases showing the classical changes in the hair coat can live happily for years before they become laminitic, diabetic or begin to lose condition. Even if the animal has suffered laminitis but in other respects appears well, these cases can be greatly improved by correct foot dressing and, or, shoeing. The precise prevalence of the neoplasm is unknown but it is probably quite common in elderly individuals. The long term prognosis is bad.

REFERENCES

Beech, J. & Garcia, M. C. (1985). *American Journal of Veterinary Research* **46**, 1941.

Eiler, H., Oliver, J. & Goble, D. (1979). *American Journal of Veterinary Research* **40**, 724.

Garcia, M. C. & Beech, J. (1986). *American Journal of Veterinary Research* **47**, 2004.

CHAPTER 9

Equine Laminitis

ROBERT EUSTACE

INTRODUCTION

Laminitis is one of the most common causes of lameness and disability of horses and ponies in this country. This article describes some of the gross pathological changes and the recommended radiographic technique and aims to provide some practical advice on treatment.

TERMINOLOGY

Laminitis is a disease caused by ischaemia of digital dermal tissues; it is not primarily an inflammatory disease, hence lamin-*itis* is a misnomer. The bond between the dermal and epidermal laminae (the interlaminar bond) is the only means of support of the distal phalanx within the hoof. If the ischaemic insult is severe enough to destroy sufficient interlaminar bonds the animal becomes *foundered*, i.e. the pedal bone moves distally within the hoof.

A *sinker* is an animal whose foot has suffered complete destruction of the interlaminar bonding and the pedal bone is totally loose within the hoof.

Frog support means providing support over the frog of the foot so that it acts as an arch support when the limb is loaded. It does not mean using such a thick frog support that the horse is forced to bear most of the weight on its frog. This will worsen the lameness in most cases. The frog should be trimmed before fitting frog supports.

CAUSES

The cause of laminitis is unknown; the following situations are known to frequently precede an attack of laminitis. Animals in these situations can thus be regarded as at *high risk* from laminitis. These situations may occur singly or in combination.

(1) OBESITY/OVEREATING

Obesity is the most common type seen in the UK. Many animals perform no work and are used as garden ornaments by people with no understanding of horse management. Horse owners are encouraged to overfeed their animals by feed companies, show judges and peer pressure. Native ponies require very little to eat and are unable to cope with fertilized cattle pasture.

(2) TOXAEMIC

Any systemic disease involving a septic or toxic focus, e.g. pneumonia, pleurisy, diarrhoea, colic (particularly following colic surgery), or endometritis can cause laminitis. Effective treatment of the initiating cause must be accomplished before improvement in the laminitis can be expected. Bacterial, viral, plant, chemical and fungal toxins have been implicated.

(3) TRAUMA/MECHANICAL

Fast or prolonged work on hard surfaces, e.g. jumping ponies in summer, racehorses on firm ground and inadequately fit endurance horses are at high risk.

Laminitis can also follow overzealous foot dressing or improper shoeing causing sole pressure. Following non-weight bearing lameness, the contralateral limb may founder.

Improper foot dressing of chronic founder type 1 cases allowing either a build-up of hyperplastic laminar horn beneath the front part of the wall or excessive heel growth leading to a broken forward phalangeal axis will lead to chronic or recurrent bouts of lameness.

(4) IATROGENIC

The administration of corticosteroid drugs to susceptible or stressed animals can be a cause. Other than treating life-threatening diseases such as purpura haemorrhagica, these drugs have no indications in equine practice in my opinion. The administration of long acting corticosteroids, such as triamcinolone and dexamethasone, to fat ponies to treat sweet itch is particularly dangerous. Even mixtures of drugs containing corticosteroids can cause laminitis. *The use of corticosteroids to treat laminitis is absolutely contraindicated.*

(5) HORMONAL

Some laminitis cases appear to be hypothyroid, although the indiscriminate use of thyroxine supplementation without testing is not recommended.

Elderly animals often develop neoplasia of the pars intermedia of the pituitary gland. This manifests as a failure to shed the hair coat in the spring, the coat becomes long and fine or matted. The animals are often polydipsic and may be diabetic. Laminitis is a common sequel to such tumours. Measurement of T3, T4 and cortisol following injection of thyroid releasing hormone is a useful test for both thyroid function and pituitary neoplasia.

(6) STRESS

Any stress such as overworking unfit horses, prolonged travelling in hot (or cold) conditions, anthelmintic treatment or vaccination may result in laminitis in some animals.

SOME MYTHS REFUTED

Drinking cold water after exercise may cause colic but not laminitis.

Allergies There is little evidence that hypersensitivities are causally related to the development of laminitis.

Pregnancy Pregnant animals can develop laminitis just as easily as barren animals.

Oestrus There may be a relationship between oestrus and laminitis in some animals; however, these cases are rare and changes in diet and management may prevent such cases.

Heat in the feet This is a *very unreliable* indicator. Foot temperature normally varies throughout the day.

Standing in streams or cold hosing Although the numbing effect of cold water may appear to make the animal more comfortable initially, prolonged cold will exacerbate vasoconstriction and further reduce dermal perfusion. It is doubtful whether hot or cold applications make a significant difference to the outcome of a case. If the owner must do something, it is preferable to use warm fomentations.

Hereditary predisposition to laminitis In this country heritability is unproven. However, families of animals often have the same owner whose predisposition to recurring poor management is certainly proven.

Laminitis does not just affect the front feet. Just the hind feet may be involved, or one foot or all the feet.

PATHOLOGICAL ANATOMY

The important features seen in a sagittal section of a normal digit (Fig. 9.1(A)) are:

(A)

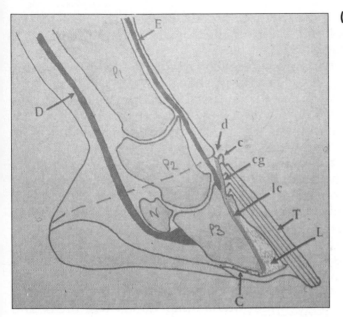

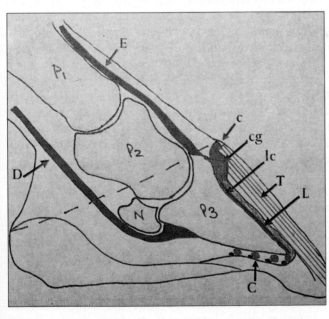

(B)

Fig. 9.1
Sagittal sections of a
normal (A) and
foundered digit (B).
P1 Proximal phalanx;
P2 middle phalanx;
P3 distal phalanx;
N navicular bone;
D deep digital flexor
tendon; E common or
long extensor tendon;
c coronary band;
cg coronary groove;
d palpable
depression just
above the coronary
band;
lc laminar corium;
C blood vessels of
the solar plexus and
circumflex artery of
the distal phalanx;
L laminae and
stratum internum of
hoof;
T horn tubules of the
stratum medium.

(1)   The top of the extensor process of the distal phalanx (P3) is slightly below the top of the dorsal hoof wall, range 0 to 10 mm (Eustace 1992a).
(2)   The coronary groove (cg) containing the coronary corium and coronary plexus is oval in shape.
(3)   The dorsal cortex of the distal phalanx is parallel to the dorsal hoof wall.
(4)   The horn tubules (T) in the dorsal hoof wall run in straight lines to the ground surface.
(5)   The solar margin of the distal phalanx is at an angle of 5° to 20° to the ground.
(6)   The apex of the trimmed frog extends dorsal to the dorsal limit of the insertion of the deep digital flexor tendon.
(7)   The horny sole is concave.

Initially during the prodromal phase of laminitis the laminae stretch resulting in a sagging down of the distal phalanx within the hoof. If the laminar insult is severe enough, or the animal is forced to walk, interlaminar bonds will break and cause further downward movement of the distal phalanx, i.e. the animal founders. The force of this downward movement is most dramatically seen in the coronary papillae. These will either be bent through an angle of up to 150° or actually be pulled out of their sockets in the epidermis (Fig. 9.2).

In the early stages of acute founder it can be seen that the "rotation" of the distal phalanx is in fact a reverse rotation of the hoof in relation to the distal phalanx. Following stretching and detachment of the interlaminar bonds, fluid extravasates into the spaces created between the dermal and epidermal laminae. The parallel relationship between the dorsal cortex of the distal phalanx and the dorsal hoof wall is lost. However the alignment of the three phalanges has not changed, i.e. there is no true rotation.

The haemorrhage and serum accumulation below the hoof wall is under pressure and creates great pain. A dorsal wall resection will remove this fluid and necrotic laminar tissue. In some laminitis cases the deep digital flexor muscle appears to go into spasm or actually shorten. It then becomes impossible to realign the phalangeal column by foot dressing. Surgical division of the inferior check ligaments or deep digital flexor tendon will be necessary.

A sagittal section of the digit of a foundered horse (Fig. 9.1(B)) shows that the coronary corium has become squeezed

(A)

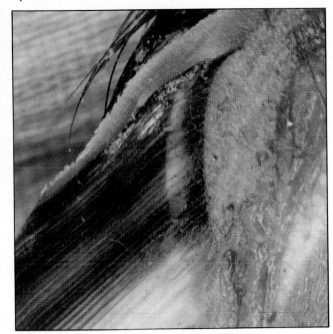

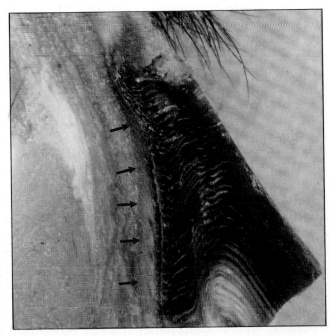

(B)

Fig. 9.2
(A) Sagittal section of a normal coronary groove and proximodorsal hoof wall. Note the curvature of the coronary groove with straight alignment of the coronary papillae pointing down the hoof wall. (B) Same region as in A of a foundered pony. The coronary groove has become less curved, the juvenile horn tubules have been bent and are pointing skywards. In this case the coronary papillae have been pulled out of their sockets in the coronary groove and have re-aligned along the line of the dorsal cortex of the distal phalanx (arrows).

between the top of the hoof wall and the front of the distal interphalangeal joint and extensor tendon (E). Unless the dorsoproximal hoof wall is thinned to relieve the compression on the coronary corium the blood supply cannot re-establish and create new wall horn. This is why untreated foundered feet have divergent growth rings with less horn formation at the toe than the heels.

Many neglected animals survive an episode of laminitis and founder to be left with the distorted feet of chronic founder. If finances preclude more effective treatments then the gait of these animals can be vastly improved by correct foot dressing and shoeing. It is important to dress the feet forward properly so as to restore the parallel relationship with the dorsal cortex of the distal phalanx. This often means rasping right through the wall proper into a mass of hyperplastic laminar horn which then shows as a buff coloured crescent at the toe of the foot (Fig. 9.3). If having dressed the foot forward there is no wall left at the toe, leaving the animal standing on its sole, a shoe must be fitted with good cover and length with upright heels and a *seated out* toe. This will prevent the animal becoming more lame.

CASE ASSESSMENT: LAMINITIS AND ACUTE FOUNDER

Palpate the digital arteries for increased volume of pulsation; increase in volume indicates either an inflammatory condition within the foot or laminitis. *Palpate the coronary bands for the presence of depressions; an abnormal depression indicates that the bone has moved due to weakening or loss of interlaminar bonding.* If a depression extends to the toe quarters, the animal has started to founder. The further back the depression can be felt towards the quarters and heels the worse the degree of founder. If the depression exists all the way back to the heels the animal is a sinker and requires immediate specialist shoeing and possibly surgical treatment within 72 hours if the animal is to have any chance of resuming an athletic career. Sinkers do not adopt the classical laminitis stance and the condition is often misdiagnosed as azoturia.

Most *laminitis* cases will respond to treatment with frog support, non-steroid anti-inflammatory drugs (NSAID),

(A)

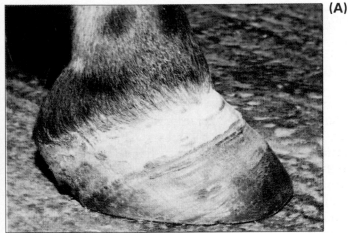

(B)

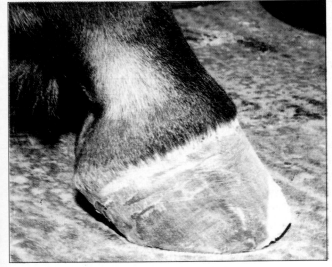

Fig. 9.3
(A) Photograph of a chronic foundered foot. Note how the toe has been "dumped" instead of dressing the foot forward properly. (B) The same foot as in A 10 minutes later. Note how the line of the most recent horn growth has been extended to the ground in a straight line. This has exposed a crescent of hyperplastic laminar horn at the toe.

phenoxybenzamine (or acepromazine as second best) and confinement in a well bedded stable. Concurrent advice on feeding and management is usually necessary.

Most *acute founder* cases will be helped by the above treatment but will require more energetic treatment (including surgical) if the feet are to be restored to functional organs.

All *sinkers* require quick and thorough treatment if they are to stand a chance of surviving.

MEDICAL TREATMENT

If the animal is sick, treat the cause. Fluids, electrolytes and possibly antibiotic therapy are indicated in cases of diarrhoea. Endometritis cases may require manual removal of retained fetal membranes followed by repeated flushing and siphoning the uterus with warm water by means of a stomach pump and stomach tube until the effluent is clear. Generally the sicker the animal the more likely it is to founder.

Phenoxybenzamine (an alpha-adrenergic blocker, unlicensed for use in equines) and heparin may be used if the animal is hospitalized and blood pressure monitoring and laboratory facilities are available. These drugs are often useful to improve digital perfusion and may prevent thrombosis in the acute case (Hood 1984). In the field, acepromazine (0.05 to 0.1 mg/kg) is a safer alpha-adrenergic blocker; it helps reduce hypertension and anxiety.

Of the NSAIDs flunixin has some analgesic and anti-endotoxic activity and may be chosen for use in sick animals. In my experience it has less analgesic effect for laminitis than phenylbutazone (4 mg/kg once or twice on the first day, reducing to 2 mg/kg twice daily) or meclofenamate (2 to 3 mg/kg once daily). Aspirin can be used singly or in combination with the other NSAIDs at a dose of 2 to 3 mg/kg once daily; it also has some anti-platelet aggregation and analgesic effects.

Blood and urine samples may be taken for full haematology, biochemistry and electrolyte examinations. Electrolyte supplementation according to laboratory results seems sensible, although in practice supplementation with chemical supplements has been unrewarding in my experience. A diet of alfalfa chop, straw chop and hay is recommended (Eustace 1992b). Supplementation with methionine (50 g/500 kg once daily and pro rata) may help liver metabolism and provides sulphur containing amino acid for horn growth. Biotin (55 mg/500 kg once daily pro rata) and zinc chelate (1 g/500 kg) are also recommended for optimal horn production (Biometh Plus; Univet). However, the product of choice is Farrier's Formula (Life Data Labs) as it is the only compound which has been shown to normalize histopathological changes in equine hoof horn (Kempson 1990). General nursing care of

very sick or lame individuals is mandatory if they are to
retain the will to live.

RADIOGRAPHIC TECHNIQUE

Lateromedial projections are the most useful. The frog of the
unshod foot is trimmed to reveal the collateral frog sulci to
their depths on both sides and around the tip of the frog. A
drawing pin with a shortened point is placed in the frog
approximately 1 cm posterior to the point of frog and its
position marked with an indelible pen or scratch line across
the sole and frog. (It does not matter exactly where on the
frog you place the pin as long as you mark its position.) The
perioplic and proximodorsal wall horn is gently rasped to
remove loose horn and create a flat dorsal surface. A straight
stiff wire marker of known length is Sellotaped to the dorsal
hoof wall. It is important to place the proximal end of this
wire where the wall horn merges with perioplic horn, i.e.
gently push the horn and place the top of the wire where the
horn starts to yield. The animal is radiographed standing
squarely on a flat wooden block incorporating a wire marker
as a ground line. The centre of the radiographic beam should
be parallel to the long axis of the navicular bone and the top
of the wooden block. The height of the beam should be such
as to show the ground line and the whole of the middle
phalanx on the developed film (Fig. 9.4).

INTERPRETATION

Accumulations of fluid cannot be visualized on foot X-rays.
Submural radiolucencies indicate the presence of gas. The
most useful prognostic criterion is the measurement of the
vertical distal displacement of the distal phalanx (founder
distance; Eustace 1992a). This is measured by drawing two
lines on the radiograph, both parallel to the ground line, one
through the top of the extensor process and one through the
top of the dorsal wall wire. Rotation of the distal phalanx in
relation to the hoof capsule is irrelevant as a prognostic
indicator. True rotation of the distal phalanx in relation to
the proximal phalanges can be of prognostic significance.

(A)

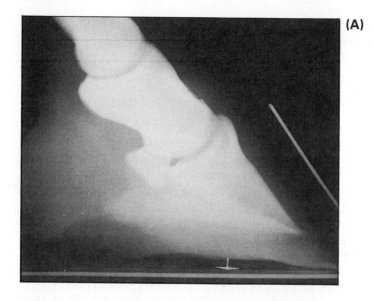

(B)

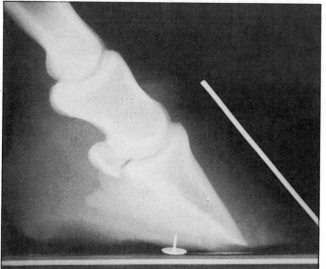

Fig. 9.4
Latero-medial radiographs of two feet. A is normal, compare with Fig. 9.5(A). B is a "sinker". Note the increased vertical distance between the top of the dorsal wall marker and the top of the extensor process of the distal phalanx. There is little true "rotation" of the distal phalanx. It is common to see a linear radiolucency along the contour of the coronary band in these cases.

Figure 9.5 shows two feet in which the angle of rotation as described by Stick, Jann, Scott and Robinson (1982) is the same; i.e. the difference in the angles between the dorsal hoof wall and the dorsal surface of the pedal bone. Figure 9.5(A) shows reverse rotation of the hoof whereas Fig. 9.5(B) shows true rotation of the distal phalanx. The foot in Fig. 9.5(A) requires either foot dressing or a dorsal wall resection. The foot in Fig. 9.5(B) requires division of the deep digital flexor tendon to effect a cure. If done before the distal phalanx becomes osteopaenic these animals often return to soundness, even if the deep digital flexor tendons in all the legs have to be divided. These figures illlustrate how meaningless it is to consider only one angle of "rotation".

The importance of recognizing and differentiating between cases of laminitis, acute founder, sinker syndrome, chronic founders type 1 and 2 cannot be overemphasized as each carries a very different prognosis (Eustace 1992a).

DOS AND DON'TS IN EQUINE LAMINITIS

Do treat laminitis with the same urgency as colic.
Do remove or treat the cause. Laminitis requires medical, shoeing and sometimes surgical treatments in combination.
Do palpate the coronary bands and provide frog support on your first visit.
Do provide the animal with a deep bed and let it lie down if it wants to.

(A)   **(B)**

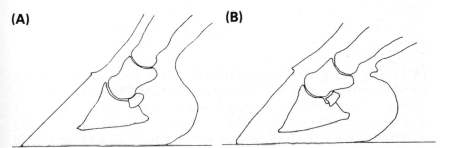

Fig. 9.5 Schematic representation of sagittal sections of two digits. A shows reverse rotation of the hoof whereas B shows true rotation of the distal phalanx relative to the proximal phalanges. The degree of rotation as described by Stick and others (1982) is the same in both parts of the figure.

Do provide frog support with either a roll of bandage, Lily pad, heart bar shoe or plastic heart bar shoe.

Do use ACP in combination with frog support. This will allow you to prescribe a lower dosage of NSAID. The toxic side-effects of NSAIDs are important, particularly in ponies and sick or elderly horses.

Do provide frog support to high risk horses. Fracture or severe sepsis cases causing non-weight bearing lameness require support on the contralateral limb. It is tedious, to say the least, to spend hours in theatre on fracture or colic cases and have them founder 10 days later!

Do radiograph the feet with markers if the animal shows the same or an increased level of pain three days after the onset of laminitis.

Do consider the relative heights of the coronary band and extensor process on radiographs. This has more prognostic relevance than "rotation" of the distal phalanx.

Do attend with the farrier if a dorsal wall resection is necessary. Although this should be a painless and bloodless procedure not requiring anaesthetic it does require veterinary supervision. Only a veterinary surgeon may perform surgery on horses.

Do consider the use of a securely fitted muzzle as a management aid in dieting ponies which can then be allowed exercise without the risk of overeating.

Do be wary of fitting heart bar shoes to animals receiving analgesic drugs; less sensitive feet cannot respond to excessive shoe pressure.

Do encourage clients to insure their horses with a reputable company against veterinary fees as hospitalization of severe cases can be expensive.

Do consider early referral of unresponsive cases.

Don't use corticosteroids.

Don't force exercise the animal. Exercise was thought to be beneficial by increasing the blood flow to the foot. There is already a tremendous increase in the blood flow to the foot but there is little or no perfusion of the dermal laminae. No amount of exercise will improve this situation and may well mechanically tear the remaining laminae, thereby worsening the founder.

Don't remove large amounts of heel from acute founder cases (including chronic founder type 1 cases suffering a secondary acute founder attack); this increases the tension in the deep digital flexor tendon and may result in more "rotation". First test by placing a wedge (equivalent in height to the amount of heel to be removed) beneath the toe of the foot and raise the contralateral limb. If the animal is more uncomfortable or if a depression appears at the dorsal coronary band, leave the heel alone.

Don't remove the shoes (other than to fit heart bar shoes) if the animal has a flat or convex sole. It will be more uncomfortable having to stand on its sole.

Don't fit any shoe other than a correctly fitted heart bar shoe to foundered horses. If the animal has foundered, the bone is loose within the hoof. The higher you raise it from the ground by means of non-support shoes, the further the bone has to move downwards.

Don't fit any device that applies pressure to the sole of the foot; it is not designed as a weight bearing structure and will easily bruise and abscess.

Don't take non-weight bearing radiographs; they are of little diagnostic value.

Don't ask farriers to fit heart bar shoes unless you have taken radiographs using markers. Good farriers will legitimately refuse to do so.

Don't forget to mark on the frog where you placed the drawing pin. If the farrier cannot appreciate where the pin was placed he is unable to fit the shoe.

Don't cut holes in the soles of laminitis or founder cases. This will result in granulating solar corium protruding through the hole which will be difficult to control. If there is subsolar fluid present, effect drainage by entering the foot through the dorsal wall at the level of the wall–sole junction. The horny sole is your biggest ally in treating laminitis and acute founder.

Don't ask the farrier to fit pads. You cannot evaluate the sole and the soles become wet due to trapped solar evaporation. Any solar pressure will further compromise the blood flow within the foot and cause pain.

Don't fight to fit shoes to horses in severe pain. There are effective glue-on alternatives available.

Don't provide repeat prescriptions of NSAIDs without revisiting. An acute laminitis case that is in significant pain after 10 days probably requires a change in treatment or management.

Don't use nerve blocks to reduce the animal's pain. The animal will further mechanically damage compromised laminae by walking on painless feet. Nerve blocks may affect the neuronal control of digital arteriovenous anastomoses and potentiate digital ischaemia.

Don't hope that antibiotics will help either "gravel" or postfounder abscesses. They won't. Only when the drainage has been provided will the lameness improve.

Don't tell the owner to starve the animal; some people take you literally. Feed according to the animal's bodily condition. Hay and bran is a poor diet for animals. If the animal needs to be dieted do so gradually using a combination of alfalfa chop, straw chop and hay. Beware of rapidly dieting very fat or pregnant ponies; they may develop hyperlipaemia which is often more serious than the original laminitis.

Don't think that because the movement of the distal phalanx has resulted in solar prolapse that is the end of the horse's working life. It is the means by which prolapse has occurred, i.e. the amount of distal displacement, which is important.

REFERENCES

Eustace, R. A. (1992a). Radiological measurements involved in the prognosis of equine laminitis. RCVS Fellowship thesis (under examination).

Eustace, R. A. (1992b). *Explaining Laminitis and its Prevention.* Bristol, R. A. Eustace.

Hood, D. M. (1984). Studies on the pathogenesis of equine laminitis. PhD thesis, Texas A. & M University, College Station, Texas.

Kempson, S. A. (1990). *Veterinary Record* **127,** 494.

Stick, J. A., Jann, H. W., Scott, E. A. & Robinson, N. E. (1982). *Journal of the American Veterinary Medical Association* **180,** 251.

CHAPTER 10

Carpal Fractures in Horses

ALISTAIR BARR

INTRODUCTION

Lameness because of carpal injury is a common cause of days lost to training in the young racehorse. Within the general heading of carpal injuries, fractures were present in 25 per cent of cases in one survey. The aetiology and pathogenesis of carpal fractures have been the subject of much speculation and suggested predisposing factors include

(1) Immaturity
(2) Conformational variations
(3) Fatigue
(4) Inappropriate foot trimming and shoeing
(5) Type of track surface

The temporal relationship between inflammatory joint disease, degenerative joint disease and intra-articular fractures of the carpus is poorly understood at present. Clinical and radiographic evidence of all three may be present at the time a horse is examined. More than one type of pathogenesis may be involved. Articular fractures may occur as a result of a single episode of overloading of a previously normal structure and give rise to an acute inflammatory response. If untreated, the combination of physical disruption of the articular surface and the release of inflammatory enzymes may result in degenerative joint disease.

PATHOGENESIS 1

Alternatively, a bone may be weakened by a pre-existing "disease" condition which increases the risk of it fracturing in response to the forces applied during "normal" activity, i.e. a pathological fracture occurs. Fractures may thus be a consequence of repetitive trauma and joint inflammation which cause weakening of the bone margin. In this situation the fracture may be regarded as a result of bone or joint disease as well as a potential cause of further joint degeneration as described above. The "disease" process involved may be physiological in origin. Bone resorption and remodelling occur in response to training with the result that the skeleton adapts to the changing forces being applied to it. During the resorption phase this process may initially weaken the bone before new bone is laid down. Subsequently sclerosis may increase the stiffness of the subchondral bone predisposing to fracture or damage to the overlying articular cartilage. In some circumstances remodelling may be too slow to keep pace with rapidly changing demands placed on the skeleton.

PATHOGENESIS 2

When these factors are taken in conjunction with the abnormal demands placed on the locomotor system of the equine athlete,

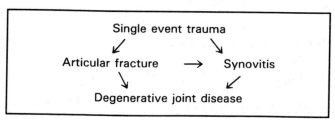

Fig. 10.1
Pathogenesis 1.

in many cases skeletally still immature, it is not surprising that carpal factures occur particularly in young racehorses.

Several different types of fracture are seen in the equine carpus:

(1) Chip fractures
(2) Slab fractures
(3) Incomplete fissure fractures
(4) Comminuted fractures
(5) Accessory carpal fractures

CHIP FRACTURES (Fig. 10.3)

Chip fractures generally affect the dorsal margins of the bones forming the antebrachiocarpal and intercarpal joints. By definition each individual chip fracture affects only one articular surface of the parent bone, although there may be multiple chips involving different bones, different joints and different limbs in the same horse.

At the time of treatment chip fractures are often accompanied by varying degrees of erosion of the surrounding articular cartilage. It is not known to what extent this damage precedes or follows the fracture itself. Clinical reports have documented varying distributions of chip fractures within the carpal joints. The most common sites in the author's experience are the

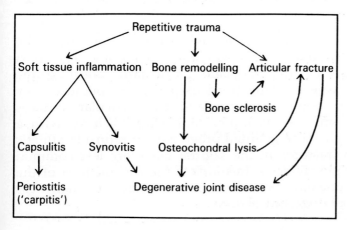

Fig. 10.2
Pathogenesis 2.

distal margin of the radial carpal bone and the proximal margin of the third carpal bone, i.e. on the dorsomedial margin of the intercarpal joint. Two biomechanical factors have been suggested to contribute to this. First, the intercarpal joint is a hinge joint where the range of motion, in full extension, is limited by contact of the opposing joint surfaces. By contrast, the antebrachiocarpal joint is a rotating joint and extension is limited to some extent by the palmar soft tissues. Secondly, the articulations between the carpal bones are so arranged that axial load is partially dissipated by horizontal displacement of the carpal bones enabling some of the load to be accepted by the intercarpal ligaments. This type of force dissipation is not, however, possible on the medial aspect of the joint where weight is transmitted directly from the radius proximally through the radial carpal to the third carpal distally.

The size of the detached bone fragment varies considerably from barely discernible flakes to pieces 1 cm or more in diameter. The fragments are often well attached to their site of origin by fibrous tissue but occasionally float freely within the joint.

SLAB FRACTURES (Figs 10.4, 10.5 and 10.6)

Slab fractures extend right through a carpal bone from the proximal to the distal articular surface. They are seen most commonly in the frontal plane particularly affecting the dorsomedial aspect of the third carpal bone. Because they involve larger bone fragments and two articular surfaces they are a more serious injury than chip fractures with a correspondingly more guarded prognosis for return to athletic activity. Slab fractures in the sagittal plane are less common but are occasionally seen. Incomplete fissure fractures of the third carpal bone have been described and may cause lameness with few localizing clinical signs.

(A)

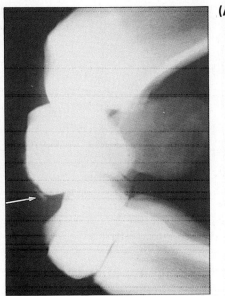

(B)

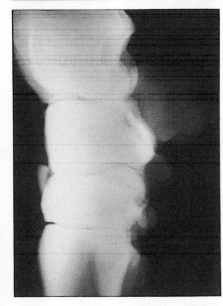

Fig. 10.3
(A) Flexed lateromedial radiograph of the left
carpus of an eight-year-old thoroughbred. There is
a small chip fracture (arrow) of the distal margin of
the radial carpal bone and irregular periosteal new
bone on the dorsal surface of the proximal row of
carpal bones. (B) Lateromedial radiograph of the
left carpus of a three-year-old thoroughbred. There
is a large chip fracture of the proximal border of
the third carpal bone.

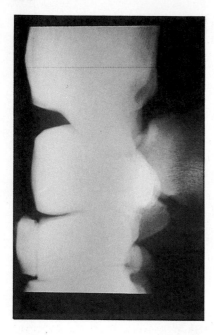

Fig. 10.4
Lateromedial radiograph of the right carpus of a four-year-old thoroughbred. There is a slab fracture of the third carpal bone.

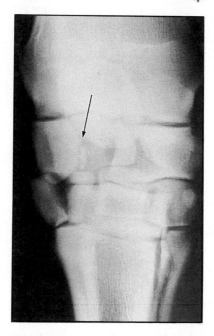

Fig. 10.5
Dorsopalmar radiograph of the right carpus of a six year old pony. There is a sagittal slab fracture of the fourth carpal bone. There is also a fracture of the distomedial aspect of the ulnar carpal bone (arrow).

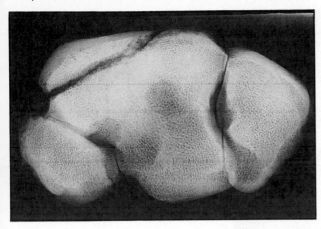

Fig. 10.6
Radiograph of a post
mortem specimen of the
distal row of carpal
bones. There is a slab
fracture through the radial
facet of the third carpal
bone.

COMMINUTED FRACTURES (Fig. 10.7)

Comminuted fractures of one or more carpal bones cause instability of the carpus and usually end a horse's athletic career. Salvage for breeding or as a pet may be feasible by a combination of internal fixation and cast support but should not be undertaken lightly. Comminution of multiple carpal bones is nearly always an indication for euthanasia.

ACCESSORY CARPAL FRACTURES (Fig. 10.8)

Accessory carpal fractures are seen most commonly in jumping horses often with a history of a fall. The fracture usually occurs in the frontal plane approximately in the middle of the bone. In the acute stage there is diffuse swelling on the palmar aspect of the carpus with palpable instability of the palmar part of the accessory carpal bone. Persistent distension of the carpal sheath may remain as the acute swelling subsides.

CLINICAL SIGNS

The degree of clinical disturbance following carpal fractures varies, depending particularly on the type and duration of

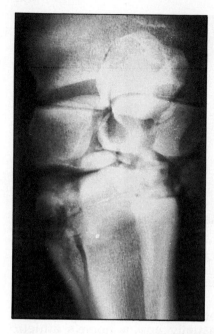

Fig. 10.7
Dorsopalmar radiograph of the right carpus of a seven-year-old partbred mare following a road traffic accident. There are multiple comminuted fractures of the carpal bones.

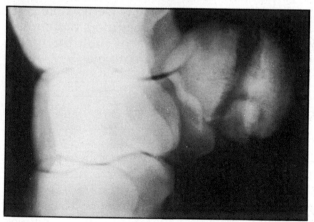

Fig. 10.8
Lateromedial radiograph of the right carpus of an eight-year-old thoroughbred. There is a frontal plane fracture of the accessory carpal bone with a large separate fragment distally.

the fractures. Animals with multiple slab or comminuted fracture will present with severe lameness and local swelling, pain, crepitus and possibly instability on manipulation of the carpus. Individual slab and sagittal fractures will show less dramatic but nevertheless pronounced clinical signs. Crepitus and instability may not be present in these cases but joint flexion is often limited. Acute chip fractures usually cause mild to moderate lameness and swelling though signs often subside with rest only to return if the animal is put back into work. Horses with chronic chip fractures that are not in work may show only mild capsular thickening.

Clinical examination should involve inspection, palpation and manipulation of the carpus in both the flexed and extended positions checking particularly for evidence of the following:

(1) Synovial effusion
(2) Thickening of the joint capsule
(3) Restricted range of joint flexion
(4) Pain on flexion or on palpation over the bone margins dorsally
(5) Palpable attached or free floating bone fragments
(6) Crepitus on manipulation
(7) Joint instability

If doubt exists as to the significance of clinical or radiological findings in relation to a presenting lameness then intra-articular anaesthesia of the antebrachiocarpal or intercarpal/carpometacarpal synovial cavities can be helpful (Fig. 10.9).

RADIOGRAPHY

Carpal fractures are not always easy to identify radiographically because the fragments may be small (e.g. many

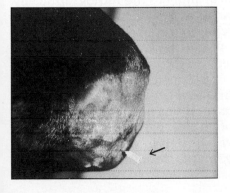

Fig. 10.9
Positioning of a needle in the intercarpal (midcarpal) joint prior to arthrocentesis or intra-articular injection.

chip fractures) or undisplaced (e.g. some slab fractures). Such abnormalities are likely to be seen only when the beam is parallel to the fracture line and the fragment is skylined. Because the exact configuration of the fracture(s) cannot be known prior to taking the radiographs the use of multiple views becomes obligatory if fractures are not to be missed. The following projections should be considered as standard.

(1) Dorsopalmar (DPa)
(2) Lateromedial (LM) (Fig. 10.10(A))
(3) Dorsolateral-palmaromedial oblique (D45L-PaMO) (Fig. 10.10(B))
(4) Dorsomedial-palmarolateral oblique (D30M-PaLO)
(5) Flexed lateromedial (Flexed LM)
(6) Flexed dorsoproximal-dorsodistal oblique (Skyline) of the distal row of carpal bones (Flexed D30Pr-DDio) (Fig. 10.11)

Both carpi should usually be radiographed as bilateral injuries are not uncommon. Because the majority of fractures seem to affect the dorsomedial aspect of the carpus, the lateromedial, flexed lateromedial and dorsolateral-palmaromedial oblique views are generally the most informative. Recent studies have emphasized the importance of the skyline view in demonstrating third carpal bone lesions. Some injuries, e.g. incomplete fissures of the third carpal bone, may be visible only on this projection. Slight variations in the degree of obliquity of particular projections may be helpful in more clearly defining lesions seen or suspected on the initial radiographs. It is important to try to relate the severity of the presenting clinical signs to the radiographically demonstrated pathological change. If there is persistent severe lameness and swelling and the radiographs show only a small chip fracture then suspicion should be aroused that a more serious injury has been missed.

Carpal fractures may be accompanied by radiological evidence of periarticular spurs of new bone suggestive of degenerative joint disease or non-articular periosteal new bone on the dorsal surface of the carpal bones ("carpitis"). The latter may be indicative of previous damage to the attachments of the dorsal ligaments linking the individual carpal bones.

(A)

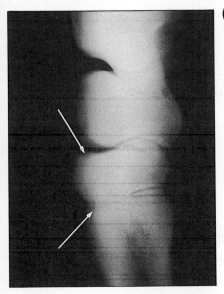

(B)

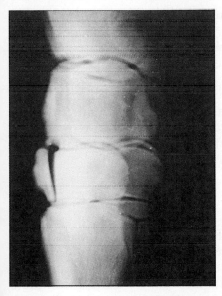

Fig. 10.10
(A) Lateromedial radiograph of the right carpus of a
five-year-old thoroughbred. A slab fracture of the
third carpal bone is just visible as a vertical line
running through the dorsal aspect of the bone
(between the arrows). (B) Dorsolateral-
palmaromedial oblique radiograph of the same
joint. The oblique view shows the slab fracture of
the third carpal bone quite clearly.

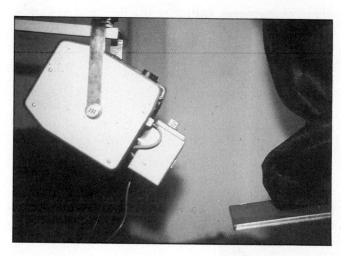

Fig. 10.11
Radiographic
positioning for flexed
dorsoproximal-
dorsodistal oblique
(skyline) projection of
the distal row of
carpal bones.

SURGERY

Surgical intervention should aim to restore articular congruency and stability and thereby minimize the development of further degenerative change within the joint. If surgery is to be performed, it is always better undertaken sooner rather than later and this in turn is dependent on early diagnosis by radiography. Surgical intervention is indicated particularly in cases of chip and slab fractures where an athletic future is planned for the horse. Chip fractures are generally treated by removing the fragment(s) whereas slabs are removed or reattached depending on their size.

CHIP FRACTURES

The advent of arthroscopy (Fig. 10.12) has allowed carpal fractures to be assessed and treated with minimal iatrogenic soft tissue damage which must be of benefit to the animal. Arthroscopy of the carpal joints also allows a more complete inspection of the articular surfaces than is possible through any single arthrotomy incision.

Initial assessment should include inspection of the articular surfaces of all the carpal bones for evaluation of the degree of fibrillation and erosion of the cartilage. The severity and extent of this damage may be as important to the prognosis as the radiologically apparent bony disruption. The synovial membrane and intra-articular ligaments may also be examined at this time. Attention is then turned to the articular margins and the fracture fragments identified. Adequate distension of the joint is vital at this stage to displace the synovial villi and allow thorough inspection of the bone margins. Fragments are frequently still attached to the parent bone or synovial membrane and must be loosened using a small elevator before being removed with grasping forceps. When all the fragments have been removed any remaining bony projections or cartilage tags are curetted smooth. The joint is then flushed through to remove any microscopic particles and drained. Single simple interrupted monofilament nylon skin sutures are then placed in the skin incisions.

Postoperatively a sterile dressing is applied to the surgical site and held in place with a heavily padded bandage. This is changed after two days and replaced with a further bandage for a week. While healing of the small skin incisions is rapid the articular surfaces take much longer to repair and a minimum of six weeks box rest followed by six weeks in a small paddock is recommended before the animal is returned to work. The rest period is extended to six months or more where there has been extensive damage to the articular surfaces.

Intra-articular medication may be helpful in promoting recovery of joint function following surgery.

Sodium hyaluronate is a glycosaminoglycan normally found in synovial fluid and articular cartilage. Among other postulated functions it is thought to act as a boundary lubricant for the soft tissues of the joint thereby promoting joint motion.

Polysulphated glycosaminoglycans are available for intramuscular and intra-articular use and have been shown to have a chondroprotective effect in experimental models of degenerative joint disease.

The effects of these drugs following surgery for carpal chip fractures are the subject of continuing investigation.

It is initially disconcerting to find that the correlation between radiographic findings and what can be seen through the arthroscope is not always good. The arthroscope often reveals considerable fibrillation or erosion of the articular cartilage around fracture fragments and on the opposing

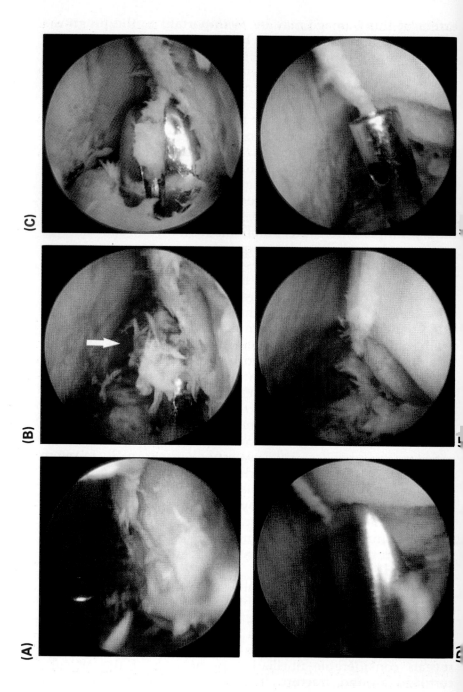

articular surface ("kissing" lesions). It may also reveal additional fragments not seen on the radiographs. Conversely, apparently separate fragments seen on the radiograph may be found to be solidly attached. While some surgeons have advocated removal of these fragments with an osteotome this is of questionable necessity in the light of the originally stated aims of surgery unless bony projections distort the normal contour of the articular surface. It is important that intraoperative decisions in this situation are based on what is best, in the long term, for the joint and not necessarily with the aim of producing a "clean" postoperative radiograph at all costs. Further clinical studies are needed to refine our understanding of the optimal approach in such cases.

SLAB FRACTURES

Slab fractures in the frontal and sometimes the sagittal plane are usually treated by screw fixation (Fig. 10.13). Initial reduction and debridement of the fracture line, where necessary, may be performed via an arthrotomy or under arthroscopic visualization. The screw is inserted in lag fashion to achieve interfragmentary compression. Even with good reduction and compression there is frequently a residual groove in the joint surface along the fracture line after surgery due to loss of articular cartilage and subchondral bone.

Fig. 10.12 The horse is in dorsal recumbency and the arthroscope has been placed into the intercarpal joint laterally between the extensor carpi radialis and common digital extensor tendons. The arthroscopic pictures therefore show the medial aspect of the intercarpal joint with the distal surface of the radial carpal bone ventrally and the proximal surface of the third carpal bone dorsally. (A) Arthroscopic view of the distal surface of the radial carpal bone. An egress cannula has been placed in the joint medially and can be seen in the top left hand corner. There is a considerable degree of full thickness erosion of the articular cartilage on the radial carpal bone. (B) The cannula is being used to push the chip fragment (arrow) up into view. There is also evidence of accompanying damage to the proximal surface of the third carpal bone seen dorsally. (C) The chip has been loosened and grasped with forceps prior to removal. (D) Loose cartilage and bone are removed with a small curette. (E) The margin of the radial carpal bone following debridement. (F) The egress cannula is used to flush through the joint and remove any small particles prior to drainage and closure.

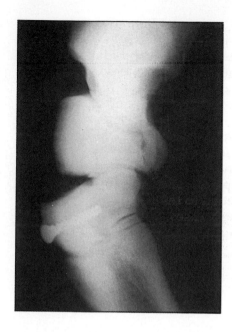

Fig. 10.13
Postoperative flexed lateromedial radiograph of the
same joint as shown in Fig. 10.10. The slab fracture
of the third carpal bone has been stabilized with a
4.5 mm diameter cortical screw.

ACCESSORY CARPAL FRACTURES

Adequate surgical stabilization of accessory carpal fractures
is difficult due to the curved shape of the bone. A degree of
communication at the fracture site is not uncommon and must
mitigate against good reduction. Both lag screw and plate
fixation have been attempted but, as with conservative
treatment, the result is usually a fibrous rather than a bony
union. Some affected horses will nevertheless be able to return
to work, including racing, despite the fracture. Those cases
where persistent lameness is associated with distension of
the carpal sheath may benefit from resection of the carpal
flexor retinaculum.

CONCLUSION

Many carpal fractures are amenable to surgical treatment.
However, surgery is liable to achieve its best results only if
performed soon after the initial injury occurs. In those cases
where chip fractures are an end product of progressive joint

disease promoted by continued work such early recognition is not always easy. Small chip fractures cause limited clinical disturbance which settles down rapidly with rest. It may be tempting to avoid or delay the radiographic evaluation of such cases until such time as the repeated recurrence of clinical signs with work makes the need for radiography obvious. By that stage further damage to the articular surfaces will have occurred and the prognosis for recovery following surgery is that much more guarded. Even where surgery is not envisaged early, diagnosis is helpful in allowing a definite recommendation to be made for a period of several months rest.

The prognosis following carpal fractures is dependent on several factors including the type of fracture, its duration and the degree of compromise of the articular surface. The latter is best assessed at surgery—while radiographs indicate the extent of the bone damage, they give little information on the degree of accompanying destruction of the articular cartilage.

ACKNOWLEDGEMENTS

The author would like to acknowledge the financial support of the Horserace Betting Levy Board with regard to a current project on aspects of equine carpal chip fractures being undertaken at the University of Bristol.

FURTHER READING

Auer, J. A. (1980). *Veterinary Clinics of North America* **2**, 81.

Bramlage, L. R. (1983) *Veterinary Clinics of North America* **5**, 261.

Bramlage, L. R., Schneider, R. K. & Gabel, A. A. (1988). *Equine Veterinary Journal* Suppl. **6**, 12.

De Haan, C. E., O'Brien, T. R. & Koblik, P. D. (1987). *Veterinary Radiology* **28**, 88.

Easley, K. J. & Schneider, J. E. (1981). *Journal of the American Veterinary Medical Association* **78**, 219.

Martin, G. S., Haynes, P. F. & McClure, J. R. (1988). *Journal of the American Veterinary Medical Association* **193**, 107.

McIlwraith, C. W. (1989). *Compendium on Continuing Education for the Practicing Veterinarian* **11**, 1287.

McIlwraith, C. W. & Martin, G. S. (1984). *Diagnostic and Surgical Arthroscopy in the Horse* (ed. C. W. McIlwraith), Goleta, CA, Veterinary Medical Publications Inc. p. 25.

McIlwraith, C. W., Yovich, J. V. & Martin, G. S. (1987). *Journal of the American Veterinary Medical Association* **191,** 531.

Ordidge, R. (1980). *Veterinary Annual* **20,** 156.

Schneider, R. K., Bramlage, L. R., Gabel, A. A., Babone, L. M. & Kantrowitz, B. M. (1988). *Equine Veterinary Journal* Suppl. **6,** 33.

CHAPTER 11

Sudden and Unexpected Death in Adult Horses and Ponies

C. M. BROWN AND THOMAS P. MULLANEY

INTRODUCTION (Fig. 11.1)

When a horse or pony collapses and dies while being observed, particularly at a public event, there is often an urgent need to explain the cause of sudden death. Equally, when a previously healthy horse is found dead, owners often wish to have the cause of unexpected death determined. These cases pose a challenge to the veterinarian, not only from the diagnostic point of view, but also because of the social, emotional and legal issues which often accompany them. One can reduce the severity of some of these issues, or avoid them altogether, if a logical systematic approach is used.

At the outset an open and frank discussion with the owner and other involved parties is often valuable. They need to know what can be done, what should be done, how much it will cost, and what the possibilities are of learning the cause of death. Most surveys of sudden and unexpected deaths in adult horses and ponies indicate that a third or more go unexplained, in spite of extensive investigations.

Many factors determine whether the deaths of these animals will be investigated. One is the monetary or sentimental value of the animal. Others are if the horse is insured or if it dies during a competition, particularly at a race course. Also, if

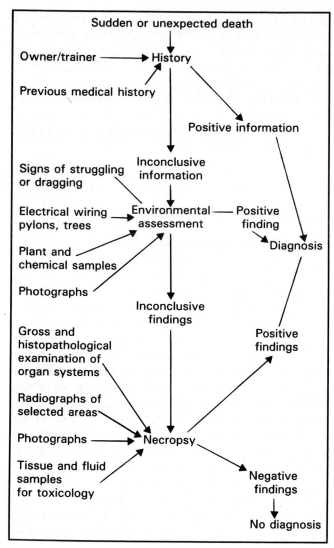

Fig. 11.1
Overview of sequences for the investigation of sudden and unexpected deaths in horses and ponies. From Brown and Mullaney (1989).

there is any suspicion of foul play, an investigation may be requested. Under certain circumstances the presence of other animals at risk may influence the need for detailed investigations. Generally speaking, the more valuable the horse, or the greater the possibility of legal action, the more likely it is that an investigation will take place.

Many horses which die unexpectedly will have died suddenly, but were not observed, and therefore were found dead. Many unexpected deaths have occurred following a clinical course of several hours, e.g. gastric dilation and rupture. Whether the deaths are considered sudden or unexpected, the overall approach to their investigation is the same. A comprehensive evaluation can be very time consuming and expensive. Owners should be aware of this from the outset. Frequently, however, valuable information can be obtained by taking a detailed history and performing a close examination of the environment.

HISTORY

Often the dead animal will have been under the care of the attending veterinarian for many years. In such cases the past medical history and management details are well known. However, some animals may have been recently acquired while others die away from home without their regular attendant present. In these cases, past medical history and management details may be incomplete. Even if present, owners and others may be too upset to communicate accurately. In other situations, people may be less than honest for fear of being considered negligent. In spite of these difficulties, as thorough a history as possible should be patiently obtained. Inconsistencies between the views of the various parties should be carefully and tactfully explored. Changes in feeding and exercise practices should be determined, and the general health of associated animals established. Recent domestic or professional disputes (e.g. the dismissal of a groom) may predispose foul play and these issues should be discussed without raising alarm. It is essential to take notes during the collection of historical information.

ENVIRONMENTAL EXAMINATION

Many horses will be seen to die suddenly or be found dead at home, but others die on the race course, show ring and hunting field. In all cases a detailed evaluation of the environment is always indicated. This should preferably be done before the horse is moved, but in public areas this may not be feasible.

Dishonest people may move a dead horse to create circumstantial evidence to support an insurance or damages claim, e.g. placing a horse under a tree after a thunder storm to suggest lightning strike, or under a power line to suggest electrocution, or in a river to suggest drowning. A careful examination should be made to determine if the horse has been dragged or carried to its current site.

Evidence of struggling in the immediate area may indicate a protracted death. Horses with severe gastrointestinal catastrophies, for example, may thrash about before dying, disturbing the surroundings in doing so, whereas electrocuted horses usually drop dead without a struggle. Others may have bled to death.

At this time, a thorough investigation for possible sources of poisons should be made. These include a wide range of chemicals and poisonous plants which may be in the feed, applied to the stable, in the water, growing in the pasture or dumped over the fence by a neighbouring gardener (e.g. yew clippings). For this reason an extensive review of the entire area may be needed. Feed and any suspicious substances should be collected into labelled containers. A photographic record of the environment may be particularly valuable, and a camera with a flash and close-up lens can be useful.

POST MORTEM EXAMINATION

If the history and environmental evaluation have not clearly indicated the cause of death, a post mortem examination must be considered. A dead horse is a bulky object and is not easily dismembered single-handed. An experienced assistant is always essential, and adequate equipment, including knives, scissors and shears is required. In most cases it may be better to transport the animal to the pathology department of a veterinary college, an investigation centre or research institute, for evaluation. This may increase the cost and delay the start of the investigation. However it may ensure a more thorough evaluation.

The post mortem examination should be as complete as possible and should not be stopped when the first lesion is found: there may be more than one cause for the animal's death. A large supply of containers, some with fixative, should be available. Sterile needles and syringes are useful for aspirating body fluids, and sterile containers may be needed for samples for microbiology.

There are many possible ways of dismembering an equine carcase, but the following approach allows for an evaluation of many organs *in situ*. Additionally, it does not require the use of hoists or ropes to support parts of the animal during the procedure. The animal is placed right side down. The external surface is closely examined and all distinguishing marks are noted, together with brands and tattoos. These may be photographed in some cases.

A ventral midline skin incision is made from the mandibular symphisis to the prepubic tendon. The skin of the left (upper) side is dissected from the body and reflected dorsally as far as possible. The left foreleg is freed of its ventral attachments by cutting the pectoral muscles and then reflected dorsally. The left hind leg is similarly reflected, and this requires incision of the capsule of the coxofemoral joint and round ligament. The abdominal wall is incised along the last rib, the ventral midline and the flank. Great care should be taken not to incise the underlying viscera. The left diaphragmatic attachments are cut. The ribs are cut dorsally and ventrally and the thoracic wall removed. Viscera are examined *in situ* and any abnormality is noted. Even if an abnormality is seen it should not be immediately removed or further evaluated. Proceed in a systematic manner.

The pelvic flexure is exteriorized and pulled ventrally. The spleen is next removed, followed by the left kidney and adrenal. The small colon is removed from the pelvic region to the transverse colon with the stump ligated with string. The small intestine is removed by stripping the organ from its mesenteric attachment. This leaves the arterial supply in place for later evaluation. The ileal stump is ligated near the caecum and duodenal stump near the stomach. The stomach is then removed. After the caecum and colon are removed the right kidney and adrenal are removed. The pelvic organs may also be removed, and this may require the pelvis to be split.

The tongue, pharynx, larynx, thyroids, trachea, lungs, heart and oesophagus are removed as a unit.

Each organ is examined separately. If no obvious causes of death are found, samples may be taken (tissues, body fluids or organ contents) for histopathology, culture, serology, biochemistry and toxicology. At least 30 g of the following should be frozen for possible toxicological examination: kidney, liver, fat, stomach contents, urine, and heart blood from the right ventricle. These samples are carefully labelled and stored until needed.

As cardiac lesions are often suspected as the cause of sudden death, particular attention should be taken to collect multiple samples of cardiac tissue to ensure a thorough evaluation of the myocardium and conducting system.

Throughout the post mortem examination, notes, either tape recorded or written should be taken. Any lesion of importance should be photographed. A written report of the gross findings should be prepared as soon as possible after the end of the examination, and selected samples submitted for further evaluation.

CAUSES OF SUDDEN DEATH

In a mixed horse population the causes of sudden death go unexplained in at least 30 per cent of investigated cases. Possible causes of sudden death, based on the systems involved are listed in Table 11.1, together with some pertinent findings.

Horses which drop dead during or immediately after a race create a rather special problem. There is often much public interest or concern, and great pressure on the attending veterinarian to explain the cause of death in a timely fashion. Foul play, usually "doping", is often suspected in the non-trauma cases. Surveys of the causes of sudden death in race horses indicate that up to 60 per cent are unexplained. However, other studies suggest that severe pulmonary haemorrhage is the major cause. Generally speaking, massive haemorrhage into the lungs, abdomen or brain is the common cause. As many of these cases of sudden death in racehorses have no obvious lesions, it is strongly recommended that the

Table 11.1 Causes of sudden death.

Cardiovascular system	
Fatal arrhythmias	Usually impossible to document based on gross necropsy findings. Presence of microscopic myocardial lesions not absolute supportive evidence as these can be found in many "normal" horses.
Acute severe myocardial necrosis	Can be associated with the ingestion of ionophore antibiotics, particularly monensin. Diagnosis based on necropsy findings and food analysis.
Rupture of mitral chordae tendinae	True prevalence not known as acute lesion may be overlooked during routine post mortem examination.
Rupture of the great vessels	Particularly in older breeding stallions as a coital or post coital event early in the breeding season. Most common site is the aortic root.
Peripheral vascular lesions	Potentially any major vessel, but frequently laceration of major hindlimb vessels following pelvic fractures. Also massive intra-abdominal or intrathoracic haemorrhage of unknown cause is reported in racehorses.
Respiratory system	
Pulmonary haemorrhage	Unknown aetiology, possibly secondary to chronic pulmonary disease, induced by severe exertion.
Pneumothorax	Apparently rare. Usually secondary to chest trauma or penetrating wounds. Easily overlooked during necropsy.
Acute pulmonary oedema, or bronchospasm, or both	Probably an anaphylactoid reaction following intravascular injection of a variety of medications. Lesions may be minimal and history is critical.
Gastrointestinal system	
Peracute colitis	An occasional animal may die suddenly when stressed without developing diarrhoea. Lesions include oedema and petechiation of the large bowel wall with fluid gut contents.
Nervous system	
Trauma	May cause skull or spinal fractures. Not all CNS trauma is secondary to fractures. Haemorrhage and nervous tissue contusions may lead to respiratory arrest and death.
Miscellaneous causes	
Lightning strike Electrocution	Evidence often circumstantial and lesions may be absent.
Gunshot	Easily diagnosed if the event was observed; if not, difficult.
Toxic chemicals and plants	Readily suspected if the animal has been closely observed and was seen to ingest the agent.

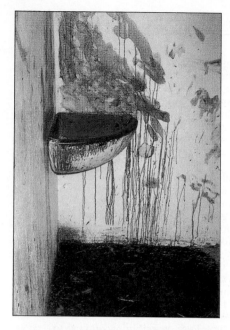

Fig. 11.2
Corner of a stall in which a horse was found dead following rupture of an aneurysm of the internal carotid artery with the guttural pouch.

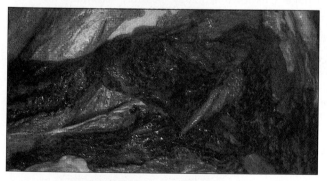

Fig. 11.3
Fatal haemorrhage within the gluteal muscles following pelvic fracture.

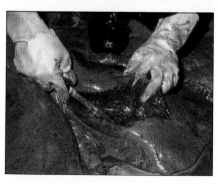

Fig. 11.4
Massive bilateral pulmonary haemorrhage in a horse which died following a race.

Table 11.2 Causes of unexpected death.

Cardiovascular system	
Vessel rupture (Figs 11.2, 11.3 and 11.4)	Medium sized vessels lacerated by trauma or fracture. Exsanguination may take several hours. Rupture of an aneurysm of the internal carotid artery, secondary mycotic infections of the guttural pouch. Middle uterine artery rupture, a post partum event in older multiparous mares. Splenic rupture, rare, usually follows trauma.
Gastrointestinal system	
Rupture of viscera	Gastric rupture. May occur following overeating of highly fermentable food or ingestion of very dry food followed by water. Also may develop when gastric motility is markedly reduced, e.g. acute grass sickness, or when there is physical obstruction to gastric emptying. Gastric ulceration may predispose to rupture. Caecal rupture: possibly predisposed by use of non-steroidal anti-inflammatory drugs. More common in post partum broodmares.
Acute enteritis	Any peracute or acute inflammatory gastrointestinal disease may lead to rapidly fatal endotoxic shock, e.g. acute salmonellosis. Post mortem findings and culture are valuable.
Anatomical derangements (Fig. 11.5)	Any displacement or bowel obstruction may lead to severe pathophysiological changes and death within hours.
Respiratory system	
Peracute pneumonia	Rarely kills within 24 hours of onset, but early signs may go unnoticed and stress or exertion may precipitate rapid deterioration and death.
Laryngeal oedema	Apparently rare.
Nervous system	
Acute meningitis	Rare.
Musculoskeletal system	
Exertional rhabdomyolysis	Severe pathophysiological changes may develop in extreme cases which are untreated. Death may ensue.
Clostridial myositis	Usually follows an intramuscular injection or penetrating wound. Most animals die within 2–3 days, but may occasionally be found dead (Fig. 11.6).

Table 11.2   Continued.

Miscellaneous conditions	
Gunshot	Deliberate shots usually involve the head or heart and diagnosis of these is straightforward.
	Accidental or deliberate chest or abdominal shots may be very difficult to diagnose. The entry site may be hidden in hair, the internal trajectory may be hard to trace, and the bullet may be lodged in a muscle belly or a viscus.
Heat stroke	Rare in temperate climates, but animals confined in poorly ventilated spaces on hot days may succumb. Post mortem findings are non-specific.
Toxic chemicals and plants	Many potential subtances, but in reality only a few are commonly encountered.

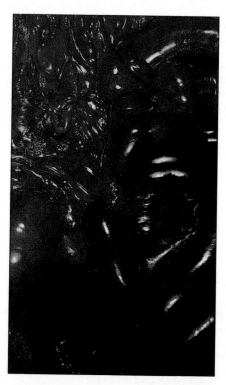

Fig. 11.5
Abdominal viscera of a horse found dead. Notice the distended discoloured small intestine which resulted from ensnarement by a pendunculated lipoma.

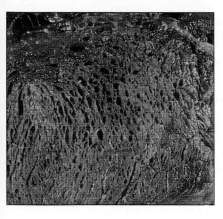

Fig. 11.6
A section of the gluteal muscle of a horse found dead as a result of clostridial myositis. The animal had received an intramuscular injection of a vitamin solution two days previously. Notice the presence of gas pockets within the affected muscle.

carcases be referred to special facilities where a thorough post mortem examination and possible toxicological examination can be done.

CAUSES OF UNEXPECTED DEATH

All of the causes of sudden death listed in Table 11.1 could also be involved in unexpected deaths. However, there are several other diseases which could have a duration of up to 24 hours before death ensues and these are summarized in Table 11.2. Again, however, it must be emphasized that at least 30 per cent may go unexplained.

TOXICOLOGICAL ASPECTS (Table 11.3)

Toxicological causes of sudden and unexpected death in horses are infrequently documented. They are, however, very frequently suspected as the cause. The range of possible toxic substances is vast. It is futile and expensive to merely pursue "poisoning" as a possible cause. Circumstantial evidence and post mortem findings must be used to guide the toxicologists as they evaluate submitted samples. It is often wise to hold samples for toxicological evaluation until all the results from gross and histopathological evaluation are available.

Table 11.3 Potentially toxic substances causing sudden and unexpected death. Necropsy findings, and samples useful for diagnosis.

Toxic substances or chemicals	Necropsy findings	Samples
Chemical toxins		
Arsenic and arsenicals	Intense hyperaemia of gastrointestinal tract, fluid haemorrhagic faeces	Liver, kidney
Chlorinated hydrocarbons	Non-specific; random petechiae	Blood, liver, fat, brain
Fluoroacetate	None	Stomach contents, liver, kidney
Monensin	Acute myocardial necrosis	Gut contents, foodstuffs
Nicotine	Non-specific	Blood, liver, kidney, gut contents
Organophosphates and carbamates	Non-specific; excess fluid in lungs and gastrointestinal tract	Blood for cholinesterase, urine, brain, gut contents
Warfarin and other anticoagulants	Massive haemorrhage into a space or viscus	Liver, kidney, whole blood
Strychnine	Rapid onset of rigor mortis	Stomach contents, liver, kidney
Plant toxins		
Black nightshade (*Solanum nigrum*)	Non-specific	Plants, gut contents to examine for poisonous plant
Caster bean (*Ricinus communis*)	Non-specific; fluid gastrointestinal contents	Plants, gut contents to examine for poisonous plant
Oleander (*Nerium oleander*)	Non-specific	Plants, gut contents to examine for poisonous plant
Hemlock (*Conium maculatum*)	Non-specific	Plants, gut contents to examine for poisonous plant
Yew	None; contaminated food often in mouth	Plants, gut contents to examine for poisonous plant
Pigweed (*Amaranthus retroflexus*) and other plants containing nitrate	Dark brownish blood and mucous membranes	Plants, gut contents to examine for poisonous plant

Modified from Brown and Mullaney (1989)

If natural substances such as insulin or intravenously administered potassium chloride are used to kill a horse, a diagnosis may be more difficult. However, immunological techniques could be used to detect if non-equine insulin is present in the carcase, while blood potassium levels may be evaluated in horses killed by an overdosage of intravenously administered potassium.

FURTHER READING

Brown, C. M., Kaneene, J. B. & Taylor, B. F. (1987). *Equine Veterinary Journal* **20,** 99.
Brown, C. M. & Mullaney, T. P. (1989). *Problems in Equine Medicine,* (ed. C. M. Brown), p. 246. Philadelphia, Lea and Febiger.
Gelberg, H. B., Zachary, J. F., Everitt, J. I., Jensen, R. C. & Smetzer, D. L. (1985). *Journal of the American Veterinary Medical Association* **187,** 1354.
Platt, H. (1982). *British Veterinary Journal* **138,** 417.
Smith, H. (1954). *Veterinary Necropsy Procedures,* (ed. T. C. Jones & C. A. Gleiser), Philadelphia, JB Lippincott.

CHAPTER 12

Practical Use of ECG in the Horse

SHEILAH A. ROBERTSON

INTRODUCTION

Electrocardiography is a useful technique in clinical equine practice for:

(1) Documenting and analysing cardiac arrhythmias
(2) Monitoring: heart rate and rhythm during general anaesthesia
(3) Studying the influence of exercise and training on the cardiac rate and rhythm of performance horses.

In man and small animals, normal electrocardiographic limits have been established for the sizes of the recorded complexes (P, QRS and T) which provide a non-invasive method of determining cardiac chamber enlargement, although dilation and hypertrophy cannot be differentiated. Since the genesis of the electrocardiogram in the horse differs from man and small animals, and because there is still a lack of generally accepted recording techniques, assessment of cardiac enlargement by electrocardiography is of little use in this species.

CHOOSING AN ELECTROCARDIOGRAPH

Numerous electrocardiographs are marketed and the choice of machine will depend on its primary intended purpose, cost and the local repair service. Some machines include facilities for direct blood pressure and temperature monitoring and unless these are required, they will add unnecessary expense.

Machines may be battery or mains operated or both. Advantages of battery operated machines include their mobility and immunity from electrical (50 Hz) interference. In addition, the animal need not usually be insulated from the ground or be earthed. Battery operated machines are less useful for long-term monitoring but can be recharged after use. When a mains operated machine is used, strict regard for electrical safety must be observed, including a machine–animal earth lead, insulation of the animal from the ground (usually by a rubber pad) and regular machine maintenance by qualified personnel.

An oscilloscope can demonstrate the ECG on a fluorescent screen. A useful feature is a "trace freeze" which prevents the waveform from moving on, or disappearing from the screen so that quick, "on-the-spot" assessments of the electrocardiogram can be made during an examination. As it is also desirable to have a permanent record of the ECG it can be recorded by connecting the oscilloscope to a direct writing apparatus (strip recorder) which can be controlled independently from the oscilloscope.

The recording paper for ECGs is normally marked in small (1 mm) and large (5 mm) boxes so that heart rates and sizes of the complexes can be calculated. Two standard chart recording speeds (25 mm/s and 50 mm/s) are often used. However, a machine with a single speed of 25 mm/s will suffice for most equine patients because of their slow heart rates. Purchasing a machine which can also run at 50 mm/s would be a worthwhile investment if it was also intended for use on dogs and cats. The faster paper speed is necessary in these species to avoid inaccuracies and cramped ECGs at fast heart rates. Figure 12.1 shows a versatile, mobile unit which can be mains or battery operated. Hospitals frequently upgrade and replace their monitoring equipment and it is often possible to purchase a suitable electrocardiograph from them

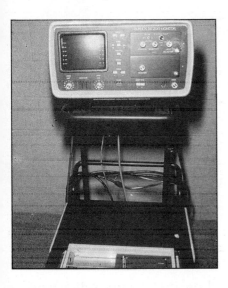

Fig. 12.1
Mobile unit (mains or battery operated) with an oscilloscope for electrocardiogram and blood pressure monitoring, and strip chart recorder for permanent recording.

at a greatly reduced cost. Obviously, these machines can only be used on a stationary horse. If electrocardiograms are desired during exercise then sophisticated radiotelemetry equipment is required. With this technique, electrodes are securely applied to the skin and a transmitter is attached to a harness or saddle.

LEAD SYSTEMS

A simple bipolar lead consists of two electrodes (one positive and one negative) which detect electrical activity in the heart from different angles. The standard limb lead system, common in small animal cardiology, results in poor quality electrocardiograms in the standing horse because of frequent shifting of limb position and muscle tremors. To overcome this problem, simple monitor lead systems have been developed for the horse.

A frequently used monitor lead is the so-called "base-apex" lead. This is recorded by attaching the right arm (negative) electrode to the left jugular furrow two-thirds of the way down the neck and placing the left arm (positive) electrode just behind the left elbow over the area of the apex beat. (This arrangement may also be used on the right side of the horse.) The ground electrode is attached at a site remote from

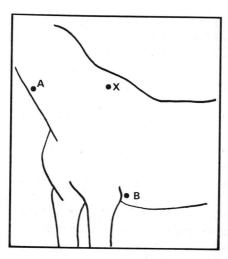

Fig. 12.2
Electrode locations for the base-apex monitor lead system. The right arm electrode (negative) is placed over the jugular furrow (A), the left arm electrode (positive) is placed just behind the left elbow over the apex beat of the heart (B). The ground electrode is attached at a site remote from the heart (X).

the heart and Lead 1 is selected on the electrocardiograph or recorder. Figures 12.2 and 12.3 demonstrate the electrode positions for the base-apex system. An alternative is the "Y" lead or the orthogonal lead system described by Holmes (1984)

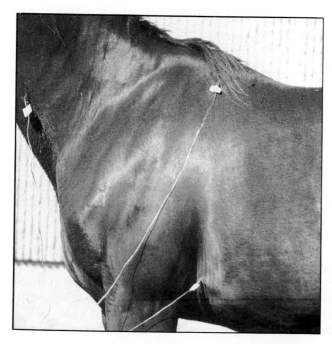

Fig. 12.3
Base-apex lead applied to a conscious standing horse using crocodile clips.

where the left arm (positive) electrode is placed over the xiphoid and the right arm (negative) electrode further cranially, over the manubrium. Again, Lead 1 is selected for recording. These monitor lead systems greatly reduce movement artefact and produce an electrocardiogram with the main QRS complex deflected downwards. A base-apex electrocardiogram is shown in Fig. 12.6. Some cardiologists prefer an upward deflection of the QRS complex so that the appearance is similar to canine and feline electrocardiograms. This can be achieved by transposing the right and left arm electrodes of the base-apex system described above, and was used to record the electrocardiograms shown in Figs 12.9 and 12.10. No matter which method is adopted, it is uniformity that is important to allow rapid and accurate comparisons between different recordings. It is also essential to note the paper speed and to know the setting of the sensitivity switch. The latter controls the amplification of the deflections and by convention a 1 mV input is set to cause the stylus to move 1 cm vertically. Once this calibration is done, the sizes of the complexes can be accurately measured.

CHOICE OF ELECTRODES AND THEIR APPLICATION (Fig. 12.4)

Silver plated electrodes are preferable to ensure good electrical conduction, but stainless steel or tin are adequate alternatives. It is important that all the electrodes are made of the same material, otherwise electrochemical currents (battery-like effect) will be created.

Artefacts are commonly encountered during ECG recording and are discussed later in this article. One of the most common causes, however, is poor electrode contact with the animal. Alligator clips are commonly used to attach the electrode tips

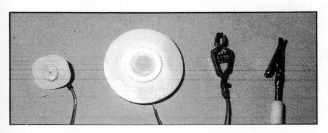

Fig. 12.4
Various types of electrodes. From left to right: paediatric and adult self-adhesive disposable patches, spring clip and alligator clip electrodes.

to the patient. These can cause tissue damage and their position should be frequently changed if used for prolonged periods. These can be made less traumatic by filing down the teeth of the clips and reducing the tension in the spring hinge.

To establish good electrical contact, the electrical resistance of the skin must be minimized and electrodes should make continuous and firm contact with the skin. Grease and dirt act as surface insulators and should be removed with acetone (10 per cent) or isopropyl alcohol. Commercial electrolyte paste and gels minimize electrical resistance and are applied liberally between the skin and alligator clips. Phisohex soap and mixtures of lubricating jelly and salt can also be used. Benzalkonium chloride and ethyl-alcohol provide good contact but, because they evaporate quickly, are only suitable for short term use. In restless foals, infiltration of the skin with local anaesthetic solution (25 gauge needle, and 2 per cent plain lignocaine) has proved to be a useful technique.

Electrode patches are available in adult and paediatric sizes and consist of a gel-filled sponge surrounded by an adhesive patch. The hair must be clipped, cleansed and thoroughly dried at the application site. Ten to 15 minutes may be required for good contact to be established because the gel must soak into the skin. These patches are not reusable, are expensive and do not adhere well if the horse is sweating, but are recommended for long term atraumatic monitoring, for example, a foal in an intensive care unit.

In the anaesthetized patient, the electrode positions may have to be modified depending on the surgical site. In surgical patients it is important that the electrodes do not dry out because access will be limited once the animal is draped. In these patients, gels and pastes can be used with conventional crocodile clips. Alternatively, sterile needle electrodes can be inserted subcutaneously or intramuscularly, taking care to minimize tissue damage.

COMMON ARTEFACTS

It is important to recognize and eliminate artefacts from the ECG recording because they may result in misdiagnosis and institution of inappropriate therapy. Common causes of artefacts are listed in Table 12.1. Electrical interference appears as a regular sequence of 50 sharp waves per second (50 Hz) making interpretation of the ECG difficult (Fig. 12.5). When these patterns are seen, ensure that the electrode clips are securely attached, have not dried out and are not in contact with each other. If electrodes have become dirty or corroded, they should be cleaned with sand paper or emery paper or replaced. Also ensure that the handler is not touching a lead, that the horse is not in contact with a wet or metal surface or has damp feet. If these measures do not eliminate the problem, unplug all other equipment in the room and/or switch off fluorescent lights. In the operating room, diathermy units may obliterate the ECG recording when in use, although some of the newer machines automatically suppress this source of artefact.

Patient movement (muscle tremors, shivering, restlessness) is less easy to resolve but will be minimized if the animal is comfortable, warm, reassured and given time to adapt to its surroundings. It is also important to have the horse standing on an even, flat surface which should be made of rubber if a mains operated machine is used. Sedation should be avoided because the commonly used agents such as xylazine and acetylpromazine may themselves influence cardiac rhythm.

A rolling up-and-down pattern or "wandering baseline" is usually caused by respiratory movements. This is usually a

---

Table 12.1 Common sources of artefacts.

Electrical interference (50 Hz)
Poor electrode contact with patient
Improper "grounding"
Other, nearby, electrical equipment
Fluorescent lighting
Patient in contact with a wet or metal surface
Damp feet

Patient movement
Muscle tremor
Shivering
Respiratory movements
Shifting stance

Interference from holder

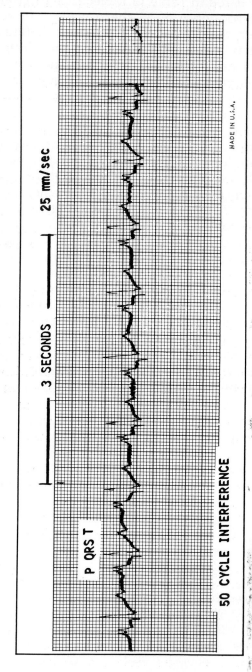

Fig. 12.5 Electrical (50 cycle) interference; the electrocardiogram cannot be as readily interpreted as usual with this artefact. Caused by inadequate electrode contact.

minor problem in a quiet resting horse but can be troublesome in an immediate post-exercise recording.

CLINICAL APPLICATION OF ELECTROCARDIOGRAPHY

It must be emphasized that the ECG is only part of the overall assessment of the patient and a good history and thorough physical examination are essential in any animal suspected of having an abnormal cardiac rhythm. Many arrhythmias are initially suspected on auscultation but may not be present continuously. Because of the intermittent nature of some arrhythmias, recordings should be made at rest, immediately after exercise and in the recovery period. Recordings can be made during exercise if, as previously described, radiotelemetry equipment is available.

The electrocardiograph only records the electrical activity of the heart and provides no information on cardiac output or tissue perfusion. This is especially important during anaesthesia because a relatively normal electrocardiogram can exist even when cardiac output is zero (electrical–mechanical dissociation). For this reason, an electrocardiograph should never be the sole means of monitoring cardiovascular function during anaesthesia. In addition, a direct or indirect blood pressure monitor, or simply "a finger on the pulse" should be utilized. As a means of counting the heart rate, the electrocardiogram can be unreliable because the tachometer in some machines will "ignore" a large downward deflection of the QRS complex which is characteristic of the horse when the base-apex monitor lead system is used.

Another clinical use of the ECG is in the assessment of changes in plasma potassium concentrations. Hyperkalaemia can produce serious arrhythmias with ECG changes first occurring at plasma levels of 6.5 to 7.0 mmol/litre and progressively worsening as plasma levels continue to rise, eventually resulting in ventricular asystole or fibrillation at levels greater than 10 mmol/litre (Epstein 1984). Foals with ruptured bladders are usually hyperkalaemic and ECG monitoring can be useful to assess their response to therapy and their suitability as anaesthesia candidates.

INTERPRETATION OF THE ELECTROCARDIOGRAM

Having mastered the technique of making a good electrocardiogram, it must be analysed to determine if it is normal or abnormal. There are numerous arrhythmias, but if a logical and systematic approach to analysis of the ECG is used, an accurate diagnosis can be made. Three basic steps will greatly simplify the process:

(1)   Calculation of the heart rate
(2)   Evaluation of the rhythm (regular or irregular)
(3)   Recognition and measurement of complexes (P, QRS and T) and their relationship to each other.

CALCULATION OF HEART RATE

First, the paper speed must be known (25 or 50 mm/s). At a paper speed of 50 mm/s, one large box is 0.10 seconds in width. When the heart rate is irregular, the approximate number of cycles (R–R intervals) between two sets of markers placed 30 boxes apart (3 seconds) can be counted and multiplied by 20 to give the heart rate/minute. When the rate is regular, the heart rate can be calculated by counting the number of small boxes between two R waves. One small box is 0.02 seconds in width, therefore, in one minute, there are 3000 small boxes (60 divided by 0.02). Thus, the number of small boxes in an R–R interval divided into 3000 gives the heart rate/minute. Figure 12.6 shows an ECG recording from a horse after exercise and illustrates how to calculate heart rate by these two methods. Equally simple mathematics can be applied for paper speeds of 25 mm/s, when one small box is 0.04 seconds and a large box 0.20 seconds. A third, quick and easy method is to use a heart rate calculator ruler (Fig. 12.7). In the resting horse, a heart rate less than 26 beats per minute (bpm) is considered to be bradycardic and a rate of over 50 bpm tachycardic.

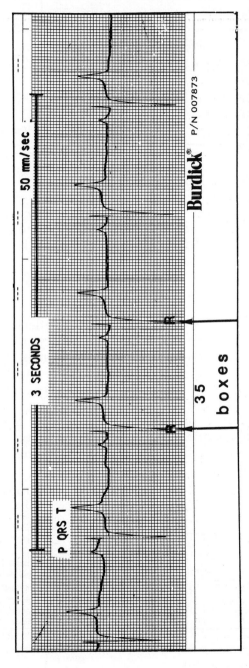

Fig. 12.6 Base-apex electrocardiogram from a horse following exercise. Paper speed is 50 mm/s. When the rhythm is irregular, the approximate number of cycles in a 3 second period multiplied by 20 gives the heart rate. In this example, 4 × 20 = 80 bpm. When the rate is regular, the number of small (0.02 second) boxes in one R–R interval (arrows) divided into 3000 equals the heart rate. In this electrocardiogram 3000 ÷ 35 = 86 bpm.

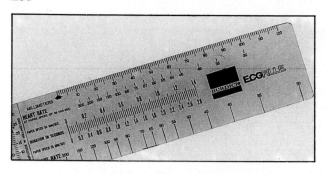

Fig. 12.7
Heart rate calculator ruler.

EVALUATION OF RHYTHM

A general inspection of the strip should determine if there is a normal (sinus) rhythm. Several sections of the strip should be studied as some arrhythmias may only occur intermittently.

RECOGNITION OF COMPLEXES

First, identify the P waves which are a reflection of atrial activity. Compare their shape and regularity. Changes in P wave shape are common in normal horses (wandering pacemaker). The configuration of the QRS complex should then be assessed. A normal QRS complex is shown in Fig. 12.8 and represents ventricular depolarization. If the QRS complex is widened or bizarre in shape, it may indicate abnormal ectopic ventricular activity. Ventricular repolarization is associated with the T wave. Also assess the relationship

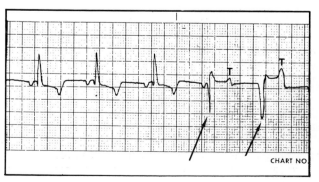

Fig. 12.8
The arrows on this tracing show ventricular premature beats or contractions (VPCs). The QRS complex of these beats are wide and abnormal in shape and followed by an opposite-polarity T wave. The two abnormal complexes have different morphology suggesting that they arise from different ectopic foci in the ventricles. Paper speed is 25 mm/s.

between the P wave and QRS complexes. Each P wave should be followed by a QRS complex and this should occur at a regular distance after the P wave. Aberrance from this pattern may indicate problems with electrical conduction within the heart. The amplitude of complexes is measured in milliseconds. Although the amplitude and duration of complexes show age, sex and breed variations these should not influence the overall interpretation of the ECG. For details of these individual changes, the reader is referred to the work of Fregin (1982). Analysis of complex arrhythmias may require the help and knowledge of an expert cardiologist but the most important part is the recording of a clear electrocardiogram with large deflections, no artefacts, and of known paper speed and calibration (1 mV = 1 cm).

CARDIAC ARRHYTHMIAS

Compared to the other domestic animal species, the horse has a higher incidence of cardiac arrhythmias, estimated to be as high as 25 to 30 per cent. However, many are considered normal and benign in the resting horse, and do not require treatment. The reason for these variations in rate and rhythm in the horse is thought to be a result of high vagal tone which has a slowing influence on heart rate and conduction. The most important consideration regarding arrhythmias in the horse is accurate diagnosis and a full assessment of the significance of the arrhythmia. Normal, "physiological" arrhythmias commonly encountered in resting horses are

Table 12.2 "Normal" cardiac arrhythmias in the horse.

Sinus arrhythmia (cyclic changes in heart rate)
Respiratory; HR increases with inspiration and decreases with expiration
Non-respiratory

Wandering atrial pacemaker (variation in shape and size of P-waves)

Incomplete atrio-ventricular block
First degree; prolonged interval between P and R complexes
Second degree; some P-waves are not followed by a QRS complex

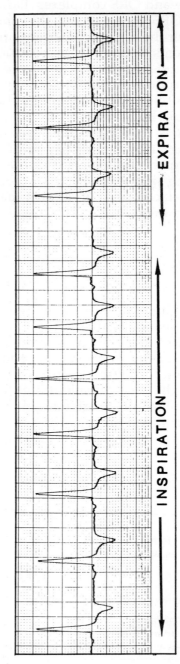

Fig. 12.9 Recording from a normal foal showing sinus arrhythmia. The cyclical increases and decreases in heart rate were correlated with respiratory activity. Paper speed is 25 mm/s.

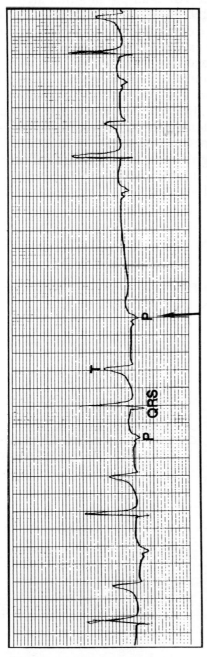

Fig. 12.10 This electrocardiogram shows second-degree atrioventricular block which is very common in normal horses. This type of block occurs when the electrical signal from the atria is not conducted to the ventricles and appears as a random P wave (arrow) that is not followed by a QRS complex. Paper speed is 25 mm/s.

listed in Table 12.2. An example of sinus arrhythmia in a foal is shown in Fig. 12.9. Figure 12.10 demonstrates a common but benign second-degree atrioventricular block in a thoroughbred racehorse. These are considered benign if they disappear in response to exercise, excitement or administration of anticholinergic agents such as atropine, all of which decrease vagal influence on the heart. This is one reason for ECG recording at rest, after exercise and during recovery.

If the simple rules outlined above are followed, one should be able to differentiate normal from abnormal equine ECGs. Discussion of significant or pathological arrhythmias are outside the scope of this paper and the reader is referred to the articles by Hilwig (1987) and McGuirk and Muir (1985).

ACKNOWLEDGEMENTS

The author thanks Dr Chris Brown for providing some of the electrocardiograms used in this article.

REFERENCES

Epstein, V. (1984). *Equine Veterinary Journal* **16**, 453.
Fregin, G. F. (1982). *Cornell Veterinarium* **72**, 304.
Holmes, J. R. (1984). *Equine Veterinary Journal* **16**, 477.
Hilwig, R. W. (1987). *Current Therapy in Equine Medicine* 2, (ed. N. E. Robinson), p. 154. Philadelphia, W. B. Saunders Company.
McGuirk, S. M. & Muir, W. W. (1985). *Veterinary Clinics of North America: Equine Practice* **1**, 353.

CHAPTER 13

Thoracic Radiography in the Horse

TIM MAIR AND CHRISTINE GIBBS

INTRODUCTION

The value of radiography in the assessment of chest diseases in man and small animals is well established but in the horse technical limitations associated with the size of the thorax have tended to preclude its use in general practice. However, with the introduction of rare-earth intensifying screens, high-speed radiographic film and an air-gap between the patient and the film, radiographs of diagnostic quality covering much of the adult horse's thorax can be obtained using relatively low-powered equipment.

RADIOGRAPHIC TECHNIQUE

In the foal complete radiographic evaluation of the thoracic cavity can be made in both lateral and ventrodorsal (VD) or dorsoventral (DV) projections, but in the adult horse the depth of tissue in the sagittal plane virtually precludes the use of VD or DV projections and radiographic examination is limited to lateral or oblique views. The large transverse size of the adult horse's chest inevitably results in loss of detail of the

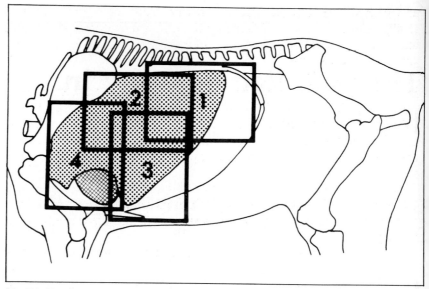

Fig. 13.1 Diagram illustrating the position of the cassette in the four different radiographic fields required for demonstrating the whole thorax of an adult horse.

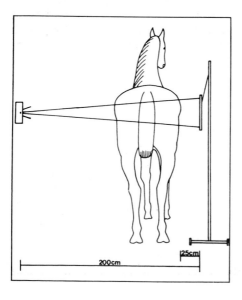

Fig. 13.2
Diagram illustrating relative positions of the X-ray tube, horse and film for thoracic radiography.

anatomical structures furthest away from the film because sharpness is lost with magnification. Therefore, if a unilateral lesion is present or suspected, radiographs should be obtained with that side adjacent to the cassette.

To avoid radiation hazards the cassette should not be held by hand so some form of mechanical supporting device is necessary. We have found that suspending the cassette in a thick cloth bag hung from a drip stand is a convenient method of achieving this. A sheet of lead 1 mm thick placed behind the cassette absorbs residual radiation and prevents back scatter.

Although the thorax of a small foal can be covered completely by a single 35 × 43 cm film, four films are usually required to demonstrate all the thoracic structures in an adult horse as shown in Fig. 13.1.

The use of an air gap between the patient and the cassette allows some of the low energy scattered radiation to be absorbed before reaching the film and eliminates the need to use a grid; this greatly reduces the exposure factors required and makes the need for absolute accuracy of centring and angulation of the cassette less critical. Figure 13.2 demonstrates

Table 13.1 Average exposure factors used at the University of Bristol for thoracic radiography (utilizing a 25 cm air gap and rare earth screens; Lanex regular; Kodak) of adult horses (450 to 500 kg bodyweight).

Machine capacity	FFD (cm)	Area of chest	mA	kVp
1000 mA; 150 kVp (Gigantos; Siemens)	200	Field 1	32–40	85
		Field 2	40–45	85
		Field 3	50	95
		Field 4	64	115
100 mA; 100 kVp (Practix portable; Philips)	200	Field 1	5	100
		Field 2	5	100
		Field 3	6	100
60 mA; 100 kVp (DX5; Philips)	100	Field 1	7	90

the system used at this centre in conjunction with a 1000 mA, 150 kV, X-ray generator (Siemens: Gigantos) and a focus-film distance of 2 m. Average exposure factors for the four radiographic fields are shown in Table 13.1. When a lower output mobile or portable unit is used, the focus to film distance may have to be reduced to 150 or 100 cm in order that the exposure time can be kept short enough to prevent motional blur. Reducing the focus to film distance has the disadvantages of reducing the amount of lung included on the side of the animal nearer the X-ray tube and increasing its distortion due to magnification.

In order to eliminate motion artefacts, the horse must be standing perfectly still when the radiograph is taken and sedation should be used if necessary. When using low-output equipment, exposure should be timed so that it coincides with a phase of respiration at which tissue movement is minimal; this is usually at end-expiration. However, if short

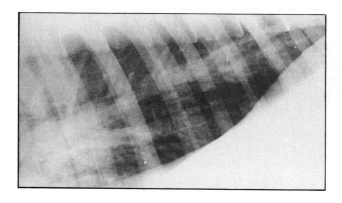

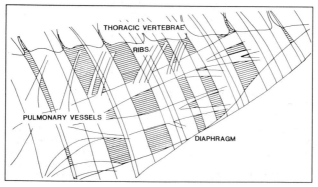

Fig. 13.3
Field 1. Dorso-caudal lung fields. Note variations in radiographic density of the lung parenchyma and the localized nodular markings which probably represent a combination of "end on" blood vessels and groups of empty "resting" alveoli.

enough exposure times can be obtained, a better quality radiograph will be produced at end-inspiration, when the lungs contain the maximum volume of air, which enhances contrast between aerated and soft tissue structures.

NORMAL RADIOGRAPHIC ANATOMY

Field 1 (Fig. 13.3) includes a large amount of lung tissue and good quality radiographs can be obtained even when low-output generators are used. Large and medium airways, pulmonary blood vessels, descending aorta, caudal vena cava, diaphragm, ribs and parts of the thoracic vertebrae can be seen in this area. The most detailed evaluation of the peripheral lung tissue and the third generation pulmonary vessels is possible here. Normal equine lung parenchyma

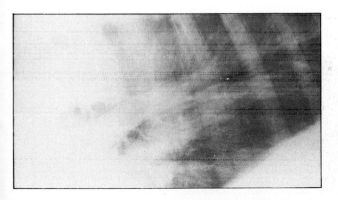

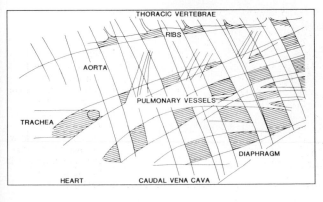

Fig. 13.4
Field 2. In this region the roots of the main pulmonary vessels, the caudal vena cava and dorso-caudal segment of the heart are included as well as a large area of lung parenchyma.

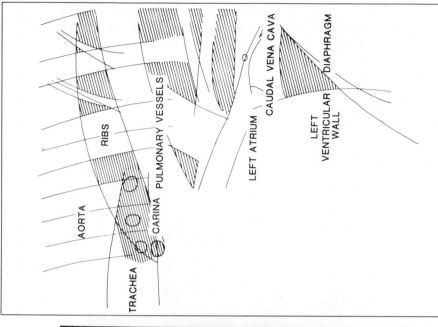

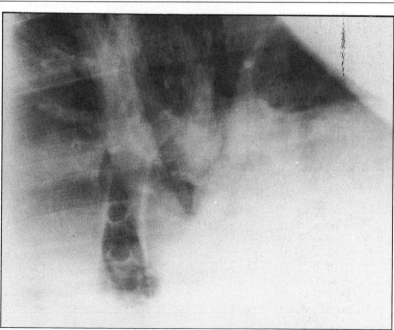

Fig. 13.5 Field 3. This area provides more information about cardiac shape and dimensions and includes the distal trachea and perihilar region. The relationship between caudal border of heart, diaphragm and caudal vena cava can be assessed in this view. Aerated lung should form an inverted triangular shape between both ventricular bor...

Labels on diagram: TRACHEA, AORTA, RIBS, CARINA, PULMONARY VESSELS, LEFT ATRIUM, CAUDAL VENA CAVA, DIAPHRAGM, LEFT VENTRICULAR WALL

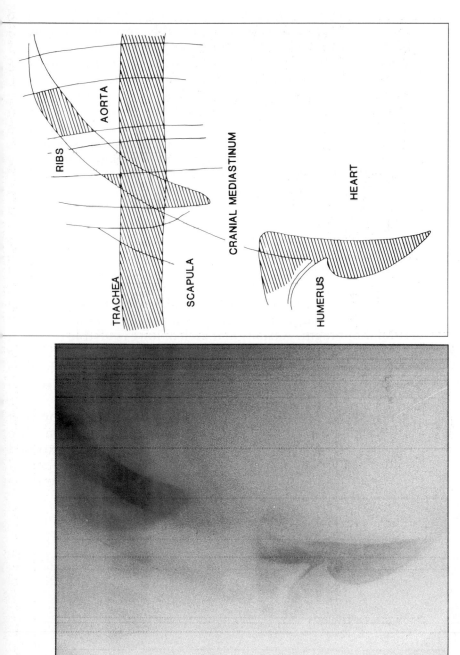

Fig. 13.6 Field 4. Only a thin "rim" of pulmonary tissue is seen between the cranial border of the heart, ascending aorta and bones of the forelimb. The cranial thoracic trachea and mediastinum can be assessed in this view.

shows a background pattern of the fine reticulo-linear and nodular radiodensities, which probably represent a combination of interstitial structures and groups of "resting" unexpanded alveoli. This appearance should not be misinterpreted as representing a pathological infiltrate.

It must be remembered that because of the domed conformation of the diaphragm, large portions of lung lateral to it will not be shown as aerated tissue. Nevertheless, gross alterations in radiodensity of thoracic contents may sometimes be demonstrated in these areas against the background opacity of the cranial abdominal contents.

Field 2 (Fig. 13.4) includes the dorsal part of the heart, the aorta, the major pulmonary arteries and veins, the distal trachea, and the carina and major bronchi. Lung tissue is more difficult to evaluate here because of the extensive superimposition of cardiovascular tissue, but the walls of the larger peripheral bronchi are occasionally mineralized and can therefore be seen as fine dense linear or ring shadows.

Field 3 (Fig. 13.5) includes the caudal part of the heart and left atrium, the larger pulmonary veins, caudal vena cava and ventral diaphragm. A triangular area of lung is visible between the heart and the diaphragm, but its precise shape and size will vary depending on the phase of respiration at which the film was exposed. The distal trachea and perihilar area can be evaluated in this region.

Field 4 (Fig. 13.6) includes most of the heart and the root of the aorta, the trachea and the cranial mediastinum. The small amount of lung tissue in this field is often overexposed because of the high factors necessary to penetrate this part of the chest, which is superimposed by the triceps muscle masses.

CHAPTER 14

Hydroponic Grass

DEREK CUDDEFORD

INTRODUCTION

Hydroponic culture is the growing of plants in a soil-less environment and has been practised for thousands of years. Water is used to transport nutrients to the plant and the major application of this cultural technique has been the production of vegetables. Hydroponically grown cereal grasses are a relatively recent innovation, their use being recorded some 100 years ago.

METHODS OF PRODUCTION

Originally the techniques for cereal grass production were fairly crude involving soaking the grain and then placing it in a warm place to germinate. Wet sacking was sometimes used as a base for the plants to develop upon as it retained water which is necessary for continued growth. In the early 1950s purpose-built growth chambers were constructed and these have been further developed and refined up to the present time.

Modern hydroponic units (Fig. 14.1) range in output from 25 to 1000 kg of fresh material/day and vary in appearance from a cloche-like apparatus to caravan-sized cabinets. Most contain a lighting system to ensure the "grass" is green as, although the nutrient content of cereal grass grown in the dark is higher than that grown in light, much of the charisma of the end product is lost if it is not green! The growth cabinets are heated to the temperature that is optimum for growth of the particular cereal that is being used. Few UK manufacturers incorporate a cooling mechanism (air conditioning) which is necessary when ambient temperatures are high (20+°C) and when the unit is in full production, as the growth process is exothermic and inadequate temperature control can lead to severe moulding problems within the unit. In addition to light and heat, there is the need to supply water to the growing material and this is usually achieved through an automatic spraying system. The water may be recycled over a 24 hour period and then replaced with fresh water. It is recommended that sodium hypochlorite is added to the water (10 mg chlorine/litre) as a hygiene precaution. Originally it was thought beneficial to add nutrients to the watering system until it was realized that the plants were too immature to take up significant quantities of nutrients.

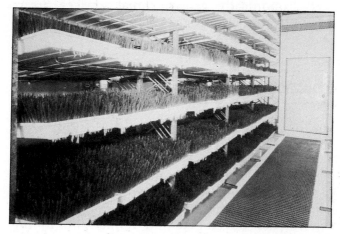

Fig. 14.1
A hydroponic unit.

PRODUCTION OF BARLEY GRASS

Barley is most often used for the production of cereal grass although any of the other cereals may be used. The optimum temperature for barley germination and growth is 20°C and the better quality thermally insulated growth cabinets are ventilated/heated/cooled to maintain this temperature ±2°C. Before introducing the high germination (>95 per cent) barley into the machine it is soaked for a minimum of six hours and preferably 12. During this period of steeping, water is imbibed by the grain and imbibation pressure ruptures the seed coat; a process known as chitting. After steeping, the chitted barley is placed in plastic trays within the growth cabinet. The whole plant consisting of roots, shoots and cereal grain residues, is used as a feed after four to eight days' growth (different manufacturers recommend different harvest times).

PHYSIOLOGY OF GROWTH

Dry barley grains contain up to 650 g starch/kg dry matter and this is the raw material which supports the growth of the plant. Imbibation of water during the steeping process activates the enzymes in the seed which hydrolyse the starch to form sugar which is available to the developing embryo. Under optimum conditions of moisture, oxygen and warmth, the sugars will be used for cell wall synthesis and to provide energy for growth. Thus the grain fuels its own growth process with a subsequent respiratory loss of dry matter. Once the shoot or plumule develops, this respiratory loss is augmented by a photorespiratory loss of carbon. The accretion of carbon through photosynthesis is very small because the light intensity in hydroponic units is usually too low and furthermore, in the immature plant, photosynthetic processes are not very efficient.

NUTRIENT PROFILE OF BARLEY GRASS

The effect of time on nutrient proportions is clearly seen in Table 14.1 (based on data obtained by Peer and Leeson 1985a).

It is apparent that there is a loss of dry matter caused by the energy reserve in the endosperm fuelling the growth process. Protein which is not used for growth will therefore increase in percentage terms but in absolute terms will remain fairly static; this will generally apply to the other nutrients. The exception is fibre which increases both in percentage and real terms because fibre is a major constituent of cell walls and structural carbohydrates, such as cellulose and hemicellulose, are synthesized. Certain vitamins such as α-tocopherol and β-carotene are produced during the growth process.

Mansbridge and Gooch (1985) demonstrated a mean increase in fresh weight yield of 500 per cent and a mean decrease in dry matter yield of 25 per cent in barley grass grown over an eight day cycle. Growth trials at the Royal (Dick) School of Veterinary Studies have shown mean dry matter losses of 20 per cent by day 5 and 23 per cent on day 8 of an eight day growth cycle. Large standard deviations are associated with these measurements and therefore individuals could experience losses greater or lesser than those given above. In this respect, it is important to realize that growing conditions and

Table 14.1 Nutrient weights and proportions of barley sprouted over a 7 day period.

	Time (days)							
	0	1	2	3	4	5	6	7
Dry matter (g)	1026	1008	996	957	902	885	867	839
Dry matter (%)	100	100	100	100	100	100	100	100
Dry matter loss (%)	—	1.7	2.9	6.7	12.0	13.7	15.5	18.2
Crude fibre (g)	55.6	56.8	59.6	55.8	66.8	86.7	94.5	119
Crude fibre (% of DM)	5.4	5.6	5.9	5.8	7.4	9.7	10.8	14.1
Crude fibre gain (%)	—	2.1	7.1	3.5	20.1	55.9	69.9	114.0
Crude protein (g)	131	128	130	131	121	123	122	130
Crude protein (% of DM)	12.7	12.7	13.0	13.6	13.4	13.9	14.0	15.5
Crude protein loss (%)	—	−2.2	−0.7	0.0	−7.6	−6.1	−6.8	−0.7

barley variety can have a large effect on the composition of the grass at any particular stage of development, e.g. increasing growing temperature to 26°C can produce grass at six days of age which has the nutrient profile of eight day grass; similarly, some varieties of barley are much more vigorously growing and as a consequence achieve an "8 day nutrient profile" earlier than other varieties. Grass produced in hydroponic units made by different manufacturers will almost certainly vary in composition even if harvested at the same age because the degree of environmental control will vary and in some machines it is inadequate.

A comparison between nutrient profiles of barley, hydroponic barley grass, and grass is shown in Table 14.2.

Of the micronutrients, the trace minerals present in the barley grass will reflect those that were originally present in the barley grain and would be present in slightly higher proportions because of starch losses. There appears to be some synthesis of vitamins (Table 14.3)

NUTRITIVE VALUE OF BARLEY GRASS

An early review (Leitch 1939) on the use of sprouted grain for livestock feeding showed that some investigators found

Table 14.2 Typical nutrient profiles of barley grass compared to barley and S23 perennial ryegrass (g/kg DM).

Nutrients	Barley grain	6 day grass (1)	8 day grass (1)	(2)	ryegrass (3)
Crude protein	112	160	186	169	159
MAD fibre	62	160	178	162*	272
Ether extract	13	22	24	23	26
Ash	30	27	28	40	75
Calcium	0.5	0.7	—	—	5.5
Phosphorus	3.9	4.7	—	—	3.2
Magnesium	1.2	1.3	—	—	1.6

*Crude fibre determined (1) R(D)SVS data
(2) Mansbridge and Gooch (1985)
(3) MAFF (1986)

Table 14.3 Vitamin analyses based on single 6 day grass samples (mg/kg DM).

Vitamin E	62.4	(7.4)
β-Carotene	42.7	(4.1)
Biotin	1.15	(0.16)
Free folic acid	1.05	(0.12)

Values for barley grain, in brackets

improvements in livestock performance whilst others observed no effect. More recent findings are given below.

PIGS AND POULTRY

Recently Peer and Leeson (1985b) showed there was a significant linear decrease (P<0.05) in metabolizable energy (ME) of dried sprouted barley with increased sprouting time (1–7 days) when fed to white leghorn cockerels. They further showed that day 4 sprouted barley was significantly (P<0.05) lower in digestible dry matter, protein and energy than ground barley although superior (P<0.05) to whole barley. Young pigs (18 kg liveweight) fed 4 day sprouted barley gained significantly (P<0.05) less weight than pigs fed on ground barley although feed efficiency was the same. These results suggest that digestibility decreases as sprouting time increases. More recent work (Cuddeford and others unpublished results) with 6 day barley grass fed to 70 kg fattening pigs has shown reductions in digestibility of dry matter (18.9 per cent), organic matter (17.6 per cent) and gross energy (20.0 per cent) of hydroponic grass compared to barley meal. The assessed digestible energy (DE) value of the barley grass was 11.72 MJ/kg DM for growing pigs.

RUMINANTS

Thomas and Reddy (1962) fed 7 day sprouted oats to dairy cows but were unable to measure improvements in milk production or milk quality. In contrast, some Russian work (Grigorev and others 1986) has shown that replacing 50 per cent of maize silage with 18 kg hydroponic barley grass increased milk yield by 8.7 per cent although milk fat was depressed.

In vitro digestibility of 8 day grass has been reported (Mansbridge and Gooch 1985) to be 0.73 and of 6 day grass to be between 0.74 and 0.72.

In vivo digestibility of barley grass in adult sheep was shown to be 0.73 by Grigorev and others (1986) and 0.76 by Mansbridge and Gooch (1985). These latter workers assess the ME of 8 day hydroponic barley grass at 12.2 MJ/kg DM.

HORSES

The digestible energy contents of 6 day hydroponic grass has been determined (Cuddeford and others unpublished results) with horses in a Latin Square experiment using different levels of grass. A mean value of 15.4 MJ DE/kg DM was obtained by difference when a basal diet of hay was fed. This value compares favourably with that of barley which is 14.5 MJ DE/kg DM for horses (Frape 1986). The digestibility of the barley grass DM was 0.74 and the grass OM was 0.77. French workers (Martin-Rosset and Dulphy 1987) showed that a concentrate composed of 59.5 per cent ground maize, 30 per cent ground barley, 80 per cent ground oatmeal and 2.5 per cent mineral vitamin supplement had a mean organic matter digestibility of 0.82 in 10 month-old horses. Thus, the value obtained for the barley grass would suggest that sprouting has had little effect on organic matter digestibility.

USES OF BARLEY GRASS

Since the late 1970s there has been a downturn in agriculture within the UK resulting in falling numbers of livestock. The most affected have been the beef and dairy sectors where numbers have fallen dramatically. In contrast, there has been an increase in sheep numbers which have utilized the land made free by the changes in other livestock enterprises. Consequently, the agricultural demand for hydroponic units in the temperate UK farming environment is low because land and grass and, or, conserved grass products are in plentiful supply. Only speciality, high value enterprises and equine units, which are almost always short of land, offer the markets for hydroponic units in the UK. However, the recent introduction of "set-aside" has made more land available for horse use and thus perhaps the market is dwindling.

ADVANTAGES

Apart from the nebulous claims made by some manufacturers, there are real advantages to be gained, although their relevance depends on individual circumstances.

LAND SHORTAGE

Having a hydroponic unit is a means of "buying" hectares as the purchase of barley seed enables the growing of forage in a very intensive fashion. To put this in context, a daily input of 200 kg barley on a 6 day cycle could yield about 1200 kg barley grass per day from a large unit which is equivalent to the daily yield of perennial ryegrass from about 2 ha at the height of the growing season.

CLIMATE

In the UK we "enjoy" extremes of climate and when drought occurs a hydroponic unit would be useful for the provision of forage. Furthermore, in extreme wet weather it would be convenient because animals could be kept off the pasture and thus prevent poaching. However, it is the seasonality of grass growth which provides a strong argument for alternative forage supplies. In-wintered/stabled animals can have continuity of grass supplies albeit in a somewhat different form.

ANIMAL HEALTH

Unfortunately winter roughages are usually dusty and now-adays many horses suffer respiratory disease making them unusable unless their feeding is very closely controlled. Barley grass presents a way round this problem and also provides a useful supplement of vitamin E and biotin.

NUTRIENT SOURCE

There can be no doubt that barley grass is valuable as a source of nutrients both in terms of energy and protein. As most roughages are deficient in protein (artificially dried legumes and grasses being exceptional in this respect) hydroponic grass can make a considerable contribution to nutrient intake, e.g. 5.3 kg hay dry matter (6 per cent protein) could be replaced by 2 kg 6 day barley grass *dry matter* (16 per cent protein) (equivalent to between 16 and 20 kg fresh material). As previously mentioned, barley grain contains a lot of starch and this contains the bulk of the energy. Cereal starches are broken down by α-amylase and α-glucosidases. Compared to the pig, which digests a lot of starch, concentrations of α-glucosidase are about the same in the horse, while the α-amylase concentration in pancreatic juice is only 5 to 6 per cent of that in the pig (Frape 1986). Thus, it is questionable how effective the horse is in breaking down cereal starch before it reaches the large intestine where large quantities can cause severe digestive disturbance. Starch is "used up" in the growth of barley grass and thus at four days about 50 per cent has been converted, at six days 70 per cent and at eight days only 0 to 10 per cent of the original starch remains. Obviously the barley grass is in a form easily digested by the horse and one can only speculate on the benefits that this may have.

PALATABILITY

Some horses show an initial reluctance to consume barley grass, possibly due to the slightly bitter taste (analogous to that of bean sprouts) but thereafter seem to find it very attractive. There can be no doubt that it adds succulence to otherwise dry winter rations and, depending on how much is fed, can moderate voluntary drinking.

EARLY BREEDING OF THOROUGHBREDS

There is circumstantial evidence to support the view that the availability of fresh green fodder (often referred to as "Dr Green") provides essential amino acids, vitamins and "other" substances which encourage early breeding.

DISADVANTAGES

LOW DRY MATTER

The mean dry matter content of the crop depends on the day of harvest; the younger the crop the higher the dry matter. Typical values determined at the R(D)SVS are given in Table 14.4.

Obviously, the nutrient density of fresh material can be low and this will limit its use in diets for high performance animals which have to be fed energy-dense feeds to minimize non-functional weight.

COST OF PRODUCTION

The capital cost of a hydroponic unit can be considerable and the quoted costs of production vary from manufacturer to manufacturer but if one takes a figure of £35/tonne, excluding

Table 14.4 The relationship between age at harvest and dry matter content of hydroponic barley grass.

Age in days	Dry matter (g/kg)
4*	187
5	155
6	125
7	115
8	107

*Not usual to harvest earlier as insufficient aerial growth.

capital repayment, then feed comparisons can be made (Table 14.5).

MOULDING

Conditions within hydroponic units are conducive to the growth of mould and the situation is analogous to the malting of barley for the brewing and distilling industries where the fungi, which occur naturally on barley, may proliferate.

Recently, Capper (1988) demonstrated the presence of members of some toxigenic species of fungi in hydroponic units although no mycotoxins were found. Adequate irrigation and routine hygiene will ensure a healthy crop of barley grass.

Table 14.5 Cost comparison between 6 day hydroponic barley grass and other horse feeds.

Feed	Costs (£)		
	/t	/kg CP	/100 MJDE
Hydroponic barley grass	35	1.75	1.86
Poor hay	70	1.75	1.00
Good hay	100	1.07	1.13
Spring cereal straw	30	1.00	0.55
Poor silage	14	1.09	0.97
Good silage	28	0.70	0.93
Grassmeal	135	0.84	1.41
Alfalfa	145	0.85	1.61
Sugar beet pulp	150	1.29	1.12
Rolled oats	180	1.99	1.44
Rolled barley	120	1.09	0.89
Wheat bran	180	1.12	1.53
Complete Horse Cubes	170	1.70	1.79
Stud Cubes	200	1.33	2.00
High Performance Coarse Mix	278	2.43	2.17
Bagged grass product	170	5.31	4.72

LABOUR REQUIREMENT

This can range from a few minutes per day to up to two hours per day with large units. Where feed is normally bought-in an additional labour requirement of this magnitude, every day of the week, can stretch resources.

CALCIUM SUPPLEMENTATION

As the grass is derived from barley, the calcium:phosphorus ratio is about 1:7 and totally imbalanced. Thus it is essential to add limestone when feeding barley grass and the amount needed depends on the desired calcium:phosphorus ratio (Table 14.6).

FEEDING BARLEY GRASS TO HORSES

The grass may be fed in mats either in racks, mangers or on the floor. Floor-fed animals are often observed placing a hoof on the mat and tearing off mouthfuls. Rack-fed animals seem to find it difficult to bite off mouthfuls and consequently shake their heads to remove the excess; this can result in waste. Probably the best way of feeding the material is to chop it and feed it in a manger by itself or mixed through the hard feed.

The size of hydroponic unit relative to the number of horses kept usually regulates the quantity of grass an individual horse receives. *Ad libitum* feeding of the grass resulted in an intake of around 60 kg by a 650 kg horse fed 3 kg long hay

Table 14.6 Limestone supplementation to achieve different calcium: phosphorus ratios.

Ca:P ratio	g/Limestone/kg barley grass DM
1:1	12
1.5:1	19
2:1	26

at the Royal (Dick) School of Veterinary Studies. We have suddenly introduced up to 40 kg of grass into the ration of 600 kg horses without any apparent ill-effect. Thus, while it is good practice to adapt horses to new feedstuffs, it appears that hydroponic barley grass may be fed at will.

We have successfully fed riding-school horses barley grass in place of conventional concentrates and these animals have worked well on a diet of hay and grass. In practice this has meant feeding about 20 kg of barley grass/day. Showjumpers, eventers, hunters and riding-school horses may be fed up to this amount divided over four feeds; obviously restricting the amount fed before work. Racehorses may be fed up to 10 kg/day although few trainers have machines big enough to produce this quantity for all their horses. Consequently in many yards there is only sufficient for an appetizer. To put this in context, 2 kg of 8 day grass will only contain about 200 g DM equivalent to 1 to 2 per cent of total intake and thus the impact on total nutrient intake will be minimal. British horses at the Seoul Olympics were fed from 10 to 15 kg of barley grass per day accounting for a minimum of 5 per cent of dry matter intake.

REFERENCES AND FURTHER READING

Capper, A. L. (1988). *Animal Feed Science Technology* **20**, 163.

Frape, D. L. (1986). *Equine Nutrition and Feeding*. Harlow, Longman Scientific and Technical.

Grigorev, N. G., Fitzev, A. J. & Lesnitskaja, T. L. (1986). *Sel'skokhozyaistven-naya Biologiya* **7**, 47.

Judd, B. L. & Matthews, J. (1974). *Feedstuffs* **46**, 25.

Leitch, J. (1939). *Imperial Bureau of Animal Nutrition (Aberdeen), Technical Communication* **11**, 3.

MAFF (1986). *Feed Composition*. Marlow, Chalcombe Publications.

Mansbridge, R. J. & Gooch, B. J. (1985). *Animal Production* **40**, 569.

Martin-Rosset, W. & Dulphy, J. P. (1987). *Livestock Production Science* **17**, 263.

Peer, D. J. & Leeson, S. (1985a). *Animal Feed Science Technology* **13**, 183.

Peer, D. J. & Leeson, S. (1985b). *Animal Feed Science Technology* **13**, 191.

Thomas, J. W. & Reddy, B. S. (1962). *Quarterly Bulletin, Michigan Agriculture Experimental Station* **44**, 654.

CHAPTER 15

Welfare Problems of the Horse

ROBERT ELLIS

INTRODUCTION

As a scientist the veterinarian finds it relatively easy to make objective opinions based on the facts available. Unfortunately welfare is an area of subjective opinion and, in the layman's mind, often tinged with emotion. Most practitioners will from time to time have been asked whether a particular case is "cruel" and the answer will probably vary from person to person. It is often easier to decide whether a case involves "unnecessary suffering". However, it is important to understand that use of such words will often involve the practitioner in legal cases concerning equine welfare. It is one thing agreeing with the crowd of bystanders that a certain case is cruel, and another appearing in court several months later to have this opinion challenged by a defence who has nothing to lose and everything to win. There is very little legislation which specifically covers welfare of the horse.

The main legislation covers those horses and ponies hired out to riders, under the Riding Establishments Acts of 1964 and 1970. These two Acts replaced an earlier Act of 1939, but are by no means satisfactory in their present state.

Licences are issued by local authorities after receipt of an application from the owner of a proposed premises and subject to an inspection by an "officer" of the authority. A licence may be issued either in provisional or full form. The officer is usually a veterinary surgeon, but this is not mandatory.

Whereas a provisional licence can have extra conditions attached to protect the welfare of the horse, the full licence does not. It is difficult to get a full licence revoked, and there is no means of withholding the licence while welfare complaints are examined.

By this means unscrupulous operators can continue to operate an establishment to the detriment of the horse. In my own experience a trekking centre managed to carry on summer operations with ponies in such poor condition that collapse was commonplace and death not unknown. It took a long time and considerable effort by the local authority and the RSPCA to bring the operator to court, after which the defendant moved his operation to the next county. Not least of the difficulties was proving that the horses were hired out, therefore, being used within the terms of the Act.

Unfortunately, these Acts only apply to a small proportion of horses in the UK; those owned, for instance, by livery yards, training yards, institutions (e.g. police), and breeding establishments are only covered by general legislation on cruelty, if at all.

How, therefore, can a veterinary surgeon arrive at an opinion in cases involving welfare which range from good, through a degree of suffering, to outright cruelty?

BASIC NEEDS

The Farm Animal Welfare Council lists five basic needs of livestock, which give a guide on the areas to be assessed (Table 15.1). However, there is no quantitative statement and the needs, therefore, are a matter of personal opinion.

Freedom from thirst, hunger or malnutrition is in itself unarguable, but the degree of malnutrition constituting "unnecessary suffering" could be difficult to define. Conversely, obesity is a welfare problem to the extent that laminitis can be a sequel. Adequate nutrition may not be easy to assess, for instance in ponies on mountain ranges,

Table 15.1 Basic needs of livestock, as assessed by the Farm Animal Welfare Council.

Freedom from thirst, hunger or malnutrition—achieved by readily accessible fresh water and a diet to maintain full health and vigour

Appropriate comfort and shelter

Freedom from injury or disease—achieved by prevention or rapid diagnosis and treatment

Freedom of movement and the opportunity to express most normal patterns of behaviour

Freedom from fear

---

although an adequate supply of water is often assumed in these cases.

Appropriate comfort and shelter can be difficult to assess for hardy types but are essential for thin-skinned horses.

Freedom from injury or disease is again arguable, but the care taken to avoid problems, and the speed at which they are tackled by the owner, are pertinent to this freedom.

Freedom of behaviour and movement can be difficult to achieve, bearing in mind that the feral horse is a creature with herd flight instinct. For the most part the horse is kept in captivity, and often in solitary confinement. It is also argued that as a herbivore, the horse is accustomed to continuous feeding, rather than a system of management more suitable for carnivores, which require shelter and intermittent feeding.

Freedom from fear cannot be gainsaid, but is difficult to quantify. Within this area the activities for which a horse is used must be considered.

STABLES (Figs 15.1, 15.2 and 15.3)

Individually stabled horses with limited or no grazing would appear, paradoxically, to be the most at risk. The sense of smell is important to the horse which has a natural tendency to form specific relationships with other horses. Possibly, therefore, most of the stable vices of weaving, crib-biting and

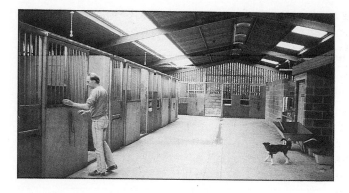

Fig. 15.1
We are used to this.

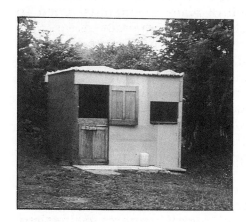

Fig. 15.2
Obviously the "Tardis" design, but check the
flooring, it may be a sea of mud.

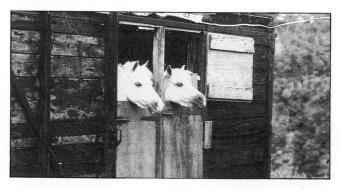

Fig. 15.3
It is dry, and they
can see out, but
watch the ventilation
when that top door is
shut.

wind-sucking are developed out of boredom and frustration. The design of the stable and level of equine activity should minimize this.

Modern stable design is poor, and ventilation inadequate, compared with pre-war stables. Shutting the top door of the stable worsens the problem, as does the habit of "mucking out" with the horse *in situ*. Such criticism is not new; earlier reports considered stables to be no more than dungeons, built with little regard for the comfort and health of the horse (Stewart 1938). The proliferation of modern wooden stabling is more a result of planning laws and cost than of welfare considerations.

The stabled horse may have limited access to grazing, both in time and space. Overgrazing in urban livery stables is still a problem today, overcrowding often forcing the horse to graze areas of pasture which it would naturally leave, thus increasing parasitism. That this is not a new problem is shown by Bartlet who in 1785 wrote, "The fields which lie near great towns, and are much dunged, are not proper pasture for horses; but on observation, appear very injurious to them, if they feed thereon all the summer".

TRANSPORTATION

All forms of vehicle are used for transporting horses. A visit to most shows or markets will reveal much to be desired. From the horse's point of view, little is known about whether there is a preference for forward facing travel as is usual, or whether the lack of vision calms or stresses the horse further.

It is perhaps of interest to a modern generation of veterinary surgeons that travelling itself killed many horses with "shipping fever" during the 1914–18 war. This acute non-contagious pleuropneumonia was overcome by removing horses with high temperatures before transport, feeding at regular intervals, and reducing time of transportation. Penning horses was found to be better than single stalling during shipping. These measures were more animal management than clinical treatment, but they improved the horses' welfare considerably.

It was noted at the same time that the veterinary surgeon should instruct the handlers in animal management, as their lack of basic knowledge created conditions suitable for disease proliferation.

The same argument could be applied today as a result of the considerable increase in the number of horse owners who have little or no knowledge of stable management. Since long distance endurance riding has become popular it has been noticed that levels of aspartate transaminase (AST) and creatine phosphokinase (CPK) can be markedly elevated without the horse showing clinical signs of azoturia. It is conceivable that these levels may relate to the travelling before the event, as the horse is often put to work soon after arriving.

POLICE WORK

Nowadays, the horse is not used for military purposes except for ceremonial use. In the 1914–18 war, over half a million horses from the UK alone were killed, although injuries from kicking, and nails in the feet were as much of a problem as enemy shells. It is doubtful if this use of the horse would be acceptable today, even if it was efficient.

However, the use of mounted police in crowd control is reminiscent of that age. While benign crowds appear to accept this use of the horse, the control of aggressive crowds leaves much to be desired. In Grosvenor Square in London (1968) rioting crowds threw marbles under the horses' feet—it is probably only a matter of time before the caltrop is reintroduced. At Hillsborough in 1988 football fans lifted a police horse off the ground by pushing underneath the animal. It says much for training that neither the horse nor rider panicked, but it does beg the question of whether the horse should be used at all for this sort of work.

COMPETITION (Fig. 15.4)

Berger (1984) argues that while there are non-competitive and competitive branches of equestrian activity, it is the competitive that has a more profound effect on breeding and selection, and the abolition of competition would hasten the horse's decline.

In this context the veterinarian should give support, but play the role of protector of the horse. Continuation of competitive activities while under the effect of drugs, for example, cannot be in a horse's best interest. So too, some of the training methods rumoured to be used in showjumping cannot be justified; for instance, closing the wings of a jump and forcing the horse out of the enclosed area. The inability of the horse to "high-jump" in an atmosphere of contrived difficulty is a popular spectator sport which leads to joint injury (Hopes 1984). To misquote Samuel Johnson, "Show jumping is like a dog walking on his hinder legs. It is not done well; but you are surprised to find it done at all".

It would be equally valid to find out whether joint disease is more prevalent in polo ponies because of the sudden changes of direction that the sport requires. Similarly, considering the damage done to young horses in the interests of racing, an increase in the minimum age for racing would be beneficial to the horse. A start could be made by moving the date at which a thoroughbred turns one year old to April, rather than January which it is at present.

The difficulty in making judgements on welfare is presented by the fact that the horse has to "earn its living". Whereas this was easy to demonstrate in warfare or transport, it is more difficult to judge with spectator sports and leisure activities.

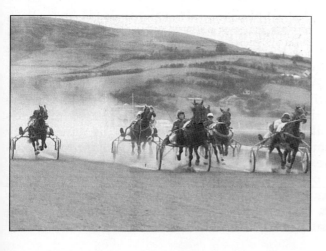

Fig. 15.4
Exciting finish, but the dust will affect the losers. Advise watering the track.

VETERINARY ROLE

As veterinarians, it is relatively easy to show the undoubted progress that has been made in control and prevention of diseases of the horse, even if the removal of veterinary curiosities peculiar to the horse, such as firing, have yet to be universally accepted. However, improvement of the horse's general welfare is still confused, partly because of the lack of "scientific" information, and partly because of lack of standards to use. Odberg (1987) elaborates on the problem, and suggests that a rider's lack of skill can stress the horse to unacceptable levels. All veterinarians must be familiar with the type of rider, who although sane on the ground, turns into Attila the Hun when on horseback!

Faced with this, it is difficult for the vet, in the role as protector, to stop the rider forcing the horse to manoeuvre in a fashion for other humans to applaud. The horse is in a position of slavery, and if incapable of performing the task, is beaten, and ultimately consigned to the saleyard.

In order to make some sense of this potential minefield what general criteria can be used by the practising vet, in assessing the welfare of a horse?

BODILY CONDITION (Figs 15.5, 15.6 and 15.7)

Bodily condition should be readily assessable by a competent vet. By virtue of seeing other horses on a regular basis, it should be possible to make a judgement on the condition of the horse, regardless of the season of the year, by comparison with its peers. While this is easier than it sounds, the difficulty arises in the witness box when what seemed obvious in the field melts in the light of cross examination. Two methods are helpful in this instance; bodyweight can be assessed by girth measurement, and, in the case of any dispute, photographs are essential.

Comparison of peer groups is essential. For instance, during the winter it is to be expected that all horses have a winter coat. However, horses with a winter coat during the spring and summer must have been short of nutrition.

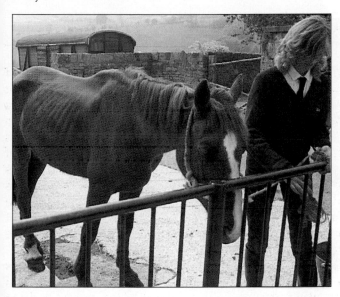

Fig. 15.5
This is unsatisfactory, either cruelty, or unnecessary suffering. NB smart outfits do not always portend well for the horse.

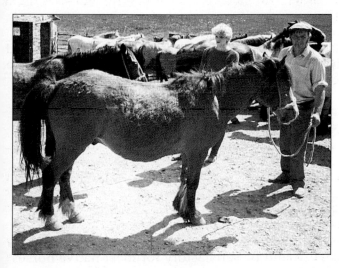

Fig. 15.6
This is hairy but fat, change of coat not complete, but condition good.

Examination of photographs will clearly show an obviously "poor" or obviously "good" horse, but what of one in between?

As a guideline, the ribs should be covered, but not have a wad of fat above the shoulder blade and the so called "poverty lines" on the rump should be absent. Thin horses, especially foals, tend to have "big heads" if poorly grown. Conversely,

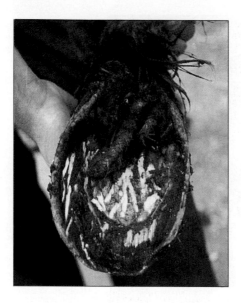

Fig. 15.7
This foot is not trimmed properly. No foot, no horse!

if a horse is in good bodily condition, the supply of water and nutrition must have been adequate.

There is also the problem of obesity in show ponies and cobs, where the fashion demands fat animals which often hover on the verge of laminitis. Here one comes up against standards laid down by show or breed societies. Persistent and patient comment to the stewards may gradually have an effect.

COMFORT AND SHELTER (Figs 15.8, 15.9 and 15.10)

Horses change their coats twice yearly. During the winter the thick winter coat should be satisfactory for most native horses not being used; however, it will be uncomfortable for a horse undergoing active exercise. Clipping therefore is commonplace, necessitating the use of rugs or housing to prevent loss of weight (condition).

Housing can consist of anything from smart stabling to railway wagons or corrugated iron lean-tos. While protection from the elements may be achieved by enclosure, it must be remembered that the horse now also needs human care to

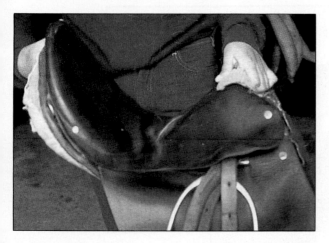

Fig. 15.8
Broken trees and homemade repairs can ruin horses' backs.

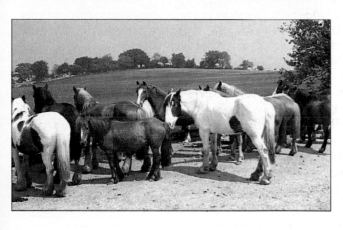

Fig. 15.9
Herds of horses are happy in close proximity if the management is good.

keep it alive. From experience it would seem that a horse is happier if it can see things going on outside the stable—as a social animal it needs companionship and will accept it from other species.

Application of the standards laid down in the Riding Establishments Acts to other situations will give some guide of the standards to be expected. Regular provision of food and water must be observed, together with exercise. A notebook and camera are essential equipment.

Estimation of available grazing should use a guideline of one acre per horse; more than this requires a strong anthelmintic "umbrella".

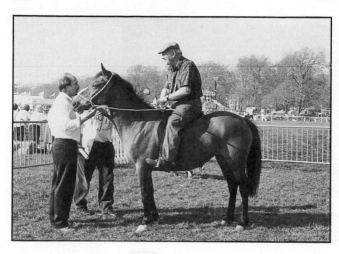

Fig. 15.10
Make sure the horse
is big enough to take
the rider.

Treatment of the horse by the rider is pragmatic. Opinion about whether the use of a riding aid is excessive will vary, but the public view today finds thrashing of a horse unacceptable, and support will be given to a veterinary surgeon who takes a sensible view. Disappointed owners tend to be vociferous in their complaints, often failing to understand that the sport in which they are involved has rules to be obeyed, whereas the spectator expects the referee to be impartial. It is better to humour the spectator.

The veterinary surgeon who is not a horseman may need courage to deal with some horseowners, but application of commonsense is normally accepted.

CONCLUSION

The welfare of the horse depends on the attitude of the human towards it. This latter has changed with the use of the horse over a period of time. Today the horse is used primarily for recreation, and there is little legislation to deal with this. It would be useful to have standards set for stabling and management, and the veterinary surgeon ought to be involved in this. A good deal of animal management is veterinary preventative medicine, and as a profession we should make sure that we are in the forefront of this. There is a natural tendency to view veterinary science as dealing purely with disease. However, the use of veterinarians in equestrian sports is a useful place to begin the education of the public. It may be necessary for some of us to be reminded of the more basic tenets in further education.

It seems unreasonable that many horses are cared for outside the framework of laws to protect them, for instance, in racing, hunting, military and police stables. Is this because these organizations have an inherited understanding of the welfare of the horse? It is important that as the use of the horse changes, so our veterinary skills look after the changing horse.

REFERENCES AND FURTHER READING

Bartlet, J. (1785). *The Gentleman's Farriery*, p. 5. 11th edn, London.

Berger, H. (1984). *Equine Veterinary Journal* **16**, 25–27.

Blenkinsop, L. J. & Rainey, J. W. (1925). *History of the Great War—Veterinary Services*.

Evans, G. E. (1966). *The Pattern of the Plough*, p. 204. London, Faber & Faber.

Ewbank, R. (1985). *Equine Veterinary Journal* **17**, 2.

Herd, R. P. & Willardon, K. L. (1985). *Equine Veterinary Journal* **17**, 235.

Hopes, R. (1984). *Equine Veterinary Journal* **16**, 1.

Jones, R. D., McGreevy, P. C., Robertson, A., Clarke, A. F. & Wathes, C. M. (1987). *Equine Veterinary Journal* **19**, 454.

Odberg, F. O. (1987). *Equine Veterinary Journal* **19**, 265.

Pollock, J. (1987). *Equine Veterinary Journal* **19**, 85.

Sainsbury, D. W. B. & Rossdale, P. D. (1987). *Equine Veterinary Journal* **19**, 370.

Soulsby, E. J. L. (1988). *Equine Veterinary Journal* **20**, 243.

Stewart, J. (1938). *Stable Economy*, 2nd edn. Blackwood & Cadell.

Wood-Gush, D. G. M. & Galbraith, F. (1987). *Equine Veterinary Journal* **19**, 129.

Index

DR CHRISTIAN'S
GUIDE TO DEALING WITH THE
TRICKY STUFF

Dr Christian Jessen

Illustrated by
David Semple

SCHOLASTIC

With thanks to Sue McMillan for her invaluable contribution
and fantastic research.

Scholastic Children's Books,
Euston House, 24 Eversholt Street,
London NW1 1DB, UK

A division of Scholastic Ltd
London ~ New York ~ Toronto ~ Sydney ~ Auckland
Mexico City ~ New Delhi ~ Hong Kong

First published in the UK by Scholastic Ltd, 2015

Text © Christian Jessen, 2015
Illustrations © David Semple, 2015
Cover photography © johnwrightphoto.com

All rights reserved.

ISBN 978 1407 15391 9

Printed and bound by Tien Wah Press SDN. BHD. , Malaysia

4 6 8 10 9 7 5 3